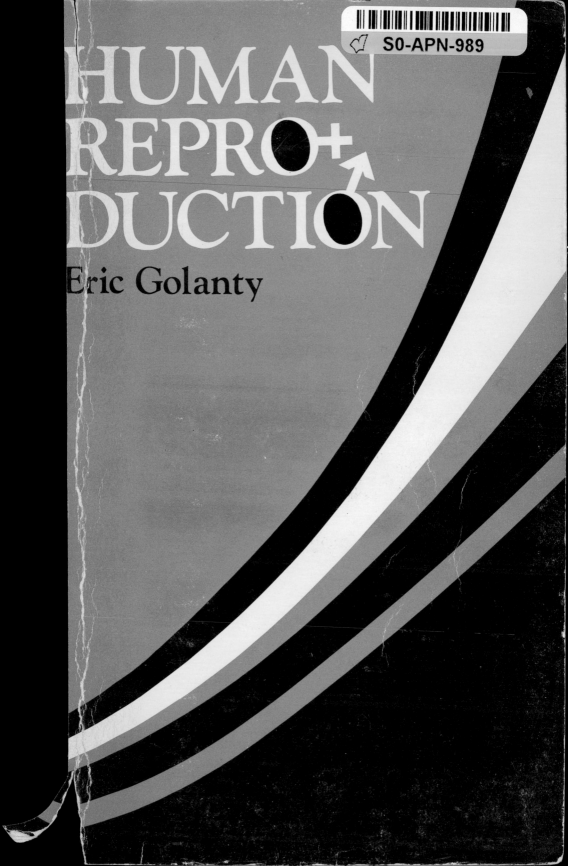

HUMAN REPRO⚥DUCTION

Eric Golanty

HUMAN
REPRODUCTION

HOLT, RINEHART AND WINSTON, INC.
*New York · Chicago · San Francisco · Atlanta
Dallas · Montreal · Toronto · London · Sydney*

ERIC GOLANTY

Instructor
Hutchins School of Liberal Studies,
California State College, Sonoma

Sex Educator
Planned Parenthood of Alameda
and San Francisco Counties

HUMAN
REPRODUCTION

Cover design: Sam Jewett
Book design: Edmee Froment

Library of Congress Cataloging in Publication Data

Golanty, Eric.
  Human reproduction.

  Includes bibliographical references.
  1. Human reproduction. I. Title. [DNLM: 1. Reproduction. WQ205 G617h]
QP251.G53   612.6   74-23202

ISBN 0-03-007001-5
Printed in the United States of America
5678   090   12345678

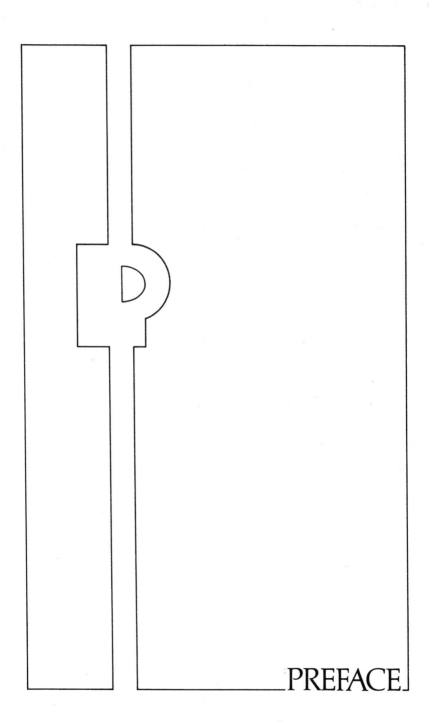

PREFACE

This book is about human sexual and reproductive biology. It is not a "how to," "when to," or "ought to" sex book. It is a biology book that contains information found in journals and monographs normally used by students and professionals in the biological and medical sciences. But it is presented here in a language and format comprehensible to the nonbiologist—without *total* dependence on a technical vocabulary and a vast array of detail. The goal of the book is to provide the reader with an intellectual framework with which to understand one of the most important facets of his or her being.

Those who teach and counsel are aware that many students and clients lack all but rudimentary knowledge of their sexual and reproductive biology. This is true despite the fact that many are sexually active and some are even parents. Moreover, their sparse accurate knowledge is usually polluted with myths and half-truths taught by parents in futile and damaging attempts to control sexual behavior. In our culture, sexual experience has never been a topic for open and honest discussion. Even with today's public display of sex, there is still resistance to open communication of sexual feelings.

Aware that they are not attaining satisfying sexual relationships, students and clients seek guidance and advice. They are eager to learn the complete truth about human sexuality and reproduction in order to become more able and fulfilled parents, spouses, and lovers.

In recent years information about human sexuality and reproduction has been liberated from the confines of the medical and psychoanalytic curriculum. Undergraduate students can take courses in human sexuality, human reproduction, and marriage and family life. Students undergoing professional training as teachers or counselors are required to master the essentials of human reproduction to perform their professional roles. Regardless of the specific course or curriculum, this book is designed to help teach the fundamentals of human sexual and reproductive biology.

Many people helped me bring this book into being, and to them I extend my deepest thanks. Deborah Doyle, Dr. Richard Strohman, and Dr. Bruce Paterson first suggested the project and encouraged me to begin. Dr. Ingrid Waldron advised me on the trials of textbook writing and helped me to find a publisher. Dr. Patricia Baker, Dr. Bent Boving, Deborah Doyle, Dr. James Ebert, Dr. David

Ehrenfeld, Dr. Garrett Hardin, Dr. William Jesse, Jo Ann Malone, Steven Robman, Patty Rosen, Dr. Sheldon Segal, Dr. Alan Sniderman, and Dr. Richard Whalen each made helpful suggestions to improve the manuscript. And Lyn Peters, my editor at Holt, Rinehart and Winston, provided the enthusiastic leadership, guidance, and support that ushered the manuscript into print.

I want to extend special thanks to Charlie, Lynnae, Steven, Alan, Debby and Tzena, whose love and support kept me going.

Eric Golanty

Berkeley
October, 1974

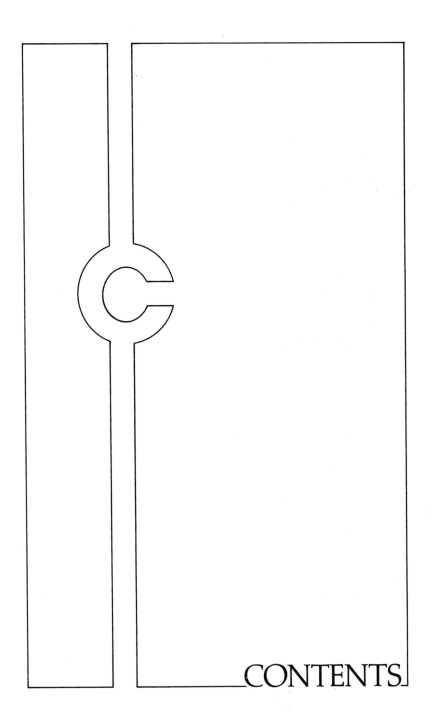

CONTENTS

CONTENTS

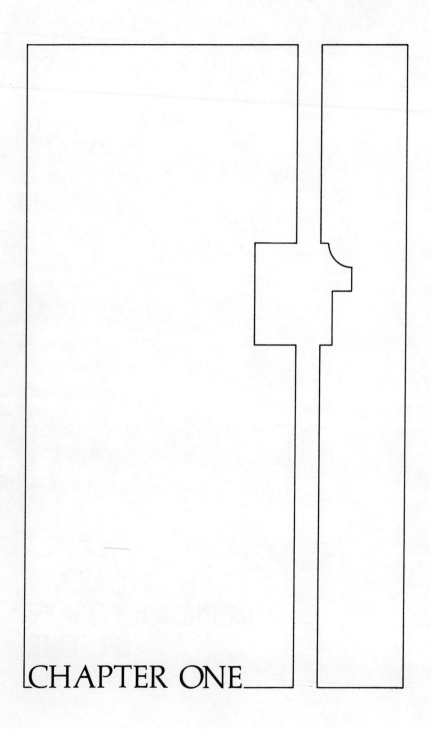

CHAPTER ONE

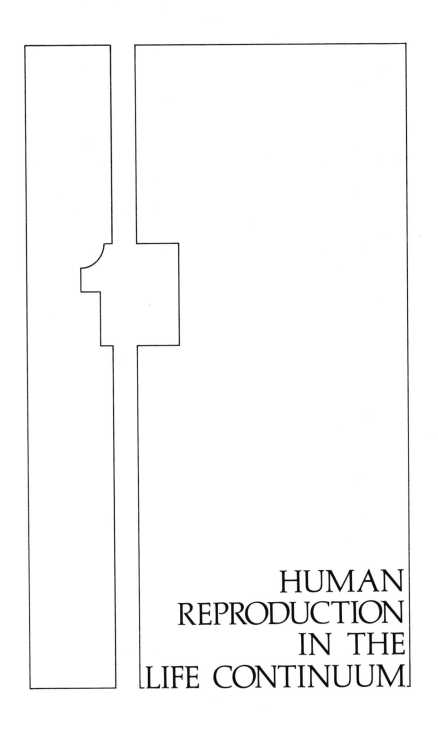

HUMAN
REPRODUCTION
IN THE
LIFE CONTINUUM

Life on earth is a continuum, which from its remote origins in the precambrian seas has maintained itself through eons of time until the present. It is unknown whether the first living things arose from the statistically improbable associations of primitive bio-organic molecules, or by colonization of the earth by primitive life forms from other regions of the universe, or by divine intervention. Whatever the originating process, the fossil evidence indicates that living things first inhabited the earth approximately three billion years ago, and from that time to this the processes of genetic variation and natural selection have produced from the original ancestral life forms the millions of species alive today as well as countless others that have already passed into extinction.

The continuation and diversification of life on earth have taken place by the production of new individuals through reproduction of already existing organisms. New organisms do not spontaneously arise from nonliving matter; they arise only from preexisting life. Because every living thing eventually dies, succumbing to disease, predation, the lethal effects of a hostile environment, or aging, life on earth continues when the individual members of a species reproduce. Reproduction compensates for losses in the species population due to death and also increases the number of individuals in the population. It fosters the continuation of that species in time.

The hallmark of organismic reproduction is the production of new living entities that are identical or nearly identical to the parent organisms from which they arise. Never do we find a plant or an animal reproducing to give rise to offspring radically different from itself. Dogs give birth to dogs and cats arise from other cats; never are kittens born to mother dogs. This conservation of organic form occurs because every generation's physical attributes are inherited from the parents. Each time reproduction occurs the parents transmit to their offspring genetic information which controls the development and function of the biochemical, anatomical, physiological, and many behavioral characteristics of the new individual. It is as if the genetic inheritance were the "blueprints" for the formation of a particular organism.

Genetic information consists of a number of discrete inheritance factors called *genes*. The genes direct the synthesis of specific proteins, which then take part in the formation and maintenance of a cell. Most proteins are enzymes—biochemical catalysts that are involved in intracellular metabolism and also in the synthesis of a cell's structural components such as membranes. Genes also carry information for the synthesis of nonenzymatic proteins, such as hormones, antibodies, and hemoglobin. Most physical attributes that we recognize as being inherited, such as eye color, hair color, body stature, and the shape of the nose, are the result of several genes acting together. These genes produce several proteins that act as a team to produce a given physical attribute.

The human genetic legacy consists of many thousands of genes, all of which are incorporated into the chemical structure of 46 threadlike *chromosomes* (Figure 1–1). As is the case with most animal species, human chromosomes occur in pairs. Twenty-two of the chromosome pairs are designated by numbers (1–22) or alternatively classified into lettered groups (A–G). The classification of the chromosomes is based upon their size and shape. The 22 numbered chromosomes are referred to as autosomes, and they are similar in every person regardless of sex. The twenty-third pair of chromosomes, however, determines the sex of the individual, and thus the members of that pair of chromosomes are referred to as sex chromosomes.

In women the size and shape of the two sex chromosomes are similar; they are designated by the letter X. The two sex chromosomes of men differ from female sex chromosomes in that they are structurally different. One of the male sex chromosomes is an X-type chromosome which resembles in size and shape the X chromosome of females. The other male sex chromosome, however, is smaller than the X and is designated by the letter Y. Therefore, the complete chromosome complement of women consists of 22 autosomal pairs of chromosomes and one pair of X sex chromosomes. Men have a chromosome complement consisting of 22 pairs of autosomes and one X sex chromosome and one Y sex chromosome.

SEX AND REPRODUCTION

The human genetic legacy is transmitted from generation to generation by the fusion of two specialized cells—a *spermatozoon*

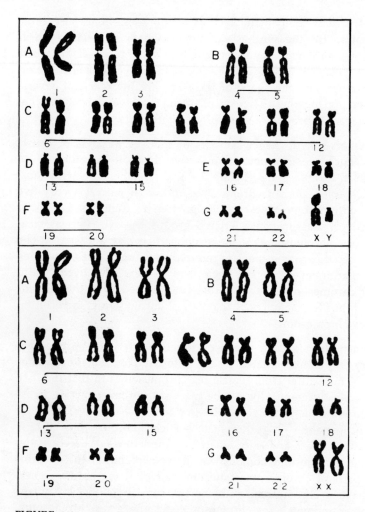

FIGURE 1-1

Chromosomes from normal male (top) and normal female (bottom) cells. From T. C. Hsu and K. Benirschke, *An Atlas of Mammalian Chromosomes*, Vol I. (New York: Springer-Verlag, 1967). Reprinted by permission.

from the father and an *ovum* from the mother (Figure 1–2). Each of these cells contains the parent's genetic contribution to its offspring in chromosomes in the cell nucleus. Unlike the other cells of the human body, the mature spermatozoon and mature ovum contain only 23 chromosomes. Although these cells originally have 46 chromosomes, they undergo a maturation process in which the

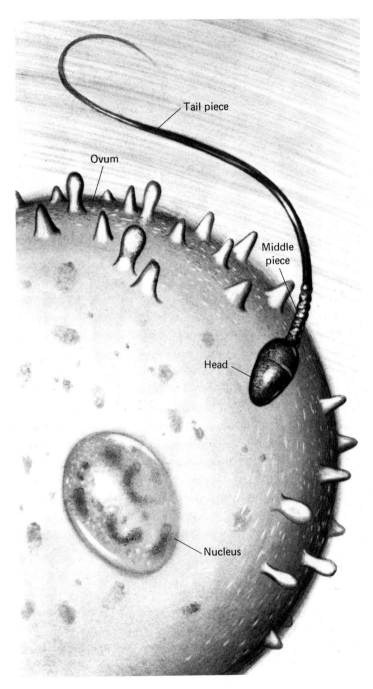

FIGURE 1-2
Human spermatozoon and human ovum.

chromosome number is reduced to 23. Therefore, when the spermatozoon and ovum fuse at fertilization the genetic contributions of both parents are brought together and the normal chromosome number of 46 is restored in the fertilized ovum.

The ovum and the spermatozoon are unique among the cells of the body, for neither of them contributes to the survival of the adult individual from which they come. Their sole function is to take part in fertilization and thereby pass genetic information from parents to offspring. The task of sustaining an individual's life is carried out by the myriad of other cells which make up the body's various tissues and organs. These cells are referred to as *somatic cells* (soma = body), whereas the sperm and ova are referred to as *germ cells* (germ = to sprout). Because they comprise the body, the somatic cells can be viewed as mere carriers of the germ cells, functioning to nurture, carry, and bring together sperm and ova so that reproduction can take place. Samuel Butler put this idea well when he said, "A hen is only an egg's way of making another egg."

Sperm have evolved as highly mobile cells, and in order to effect fertilization the sperm generally swim to ova. In animal species that reproduce in water both sexes simultaneously release thousands of gametes into the surrounding aqueous environment and fertilization occurs when spermatozoa swim toward and penetrate the relatively immobile ova. This form of fertilization is called external fertilization since it takes place outside of the bodies of the mating partners.

The fertilization process common to terrestrial animals is referred to as *internal fertilization*. It involves the actual deposition of sperm inside the body of the female. Internal fertilization in many animals including man is mediated by the joining of an outward extension of the male, called the *penis*, with an inward channel of the female, called the *vagina*. When the penis is inserted into the vagina, a tubelike path is formed leading from the male's testes, where sperm are formed, to the female reproductive tract, where fertilization takes place (Figure 1–3). The tubelike path is made up of a series of sperm ducts that lead from the testes to the penis, from the connected penis and vagina to the uterus and uterine tubes of the female. Fertilization takes place in the uterine tubes.

Internal fertilization is a more efficient reproductive mechanism

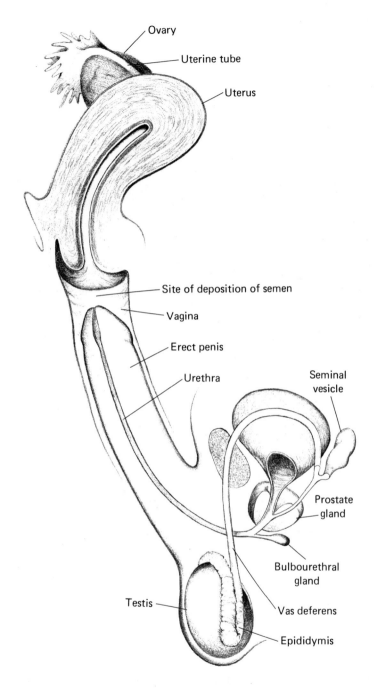

Ovary

Uterine tube

Uterus

Site of deposition of semen

Vagina

Erect penis

Urethra

Seminal vesicle

Prostate gland

Bulbourethral gland

Testis

Vas deferens

Epididymis

FIGURE 1-3
Joined male and female reproductive tracts (at coitus). Spermatozoa formed in the testes move through the two duct systems to fertilize an ovum in the uterine tube.

than external fertilization because the gametes are not released into the open environment. In animal species in which sperm and ova are spawned into open water, fertilization occurs only if there is a fortuitous collision between a spermatozoon and an ovum. So, if the male and female are far apart when they mate, or if the release of gametes takes place during bad weather, fertilization may not occur at all. Internal fertilization increases the probability of successful fertilization because the sperm are released inside the female reproductive tract in close proximity to ova, and therefore environmental factors cannot deter the rendezvous of sperm and ovum.

The involvement of a spermatozoon and an ovum in the creation of a new generation of offspring is an example of *sexual reproduction*. In sexual reproduction the two mature, fusing sex cells are referred to as gametes and their fusion produces a single cell called a zygote. In some species of lower organisms, the gametes may not be visibly distinguishable. The male gamete and female gamete are oval and appear identical. In the higher forms such as man, the male gamete is the characteristic tadpolelike cell and the ovum is usually oval or round.

Sexual reproduction is not the exclusive mode of reproduction in the biological world. Many unicellular organisms such as bacteria and other protozoa reproduce simply by splitting in two—a process known as *fission*. Where there was one cell before fission there are two cells afterward (Figure 1–4). Before fission takes place an exact duplicate of the organism's genetic material (often only a single

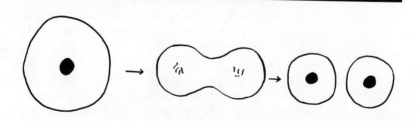

FIGURE 1-4
Asexual reproduction by binary fission.

chromosome) is synthesized in the cell so that the genetic information in the parent cell can be transmitted to each of the daughter cells produced by division. Since the genetic composition of the two daughter cells is identical to that of the parent cell, the morphology and physiology of the offspring and the parent cell are identical. This form of reproduction is termed asexual because it requires only one cell to give rise to a new generation.

Sexual reproduction provides great survival advantages for a species because it brings about variation in the physical traits of the young and thereby increases the probability that some offspring, presumably the best suited for their environment, will survive. This is not a trivial point, for when all the offspring are exact replicas of the parents, as in asexual modes of reproduction, any change in environmental conditions such that the parents cannot survive is also lethal to their young. In these instances the entire species can be destroyed. Because offspring of sexually reproducing parents inherit genes from two individuals and not just one, they are genetically and hence physically unique from their parents and other members of their species. When the progeny are in some ways different from their parents, no matter how slight the difference may be, they might be able to survive environmental changes that are lethal to their parents.

CARE OF
THE YOUNG

In order for reproduction to be successful a certain number of offspring must survive to reproduce. If the young do not survive to reproductive age or are in some other way prevented from reproducing, then the continuation of their genetic line will come to an end. The reproductive mechanisms of some animal species ensure that enough young will survive to reproduce through the production of many new offspring, often thousands at a time, so that attrition of their number by predation, disease, or other environmental hazards will leave a few, perhaps those best suited to their environment, to survive and reproduce. Other animals produce a few offspring at a time, but protect them in some way during the embryonic, and therefore most vulnerable, phase of life. In this way the chance of survival of the young is increased.

In most mammalian species including man the embryo develops inside the mother's body enclosed in a maternal organ called the *uterus*. The function of the uterus is to provide a nutritive and protective environment for the fetus as it develops from a single-celled zygote, formed by the fusion of a spermatozoon and an ovum to a multicelled infant capable of some degree of self-maintenance in the outside world. To develop inside the mother's body during the period of fetal growth is a distinct advantage, for the fetus benefits from its mother's ability to protect herself, to gather food, and to maintain a relatively constant physical and biochemical internal environment. After the period of intrauterine development the fetus is expelled from the mother's body and life in the outside world begins.

Although the newborn young of most mammalian species are capable of many life-supporting physiological functions such as breathing, digesting, eliminating waste, and sensing a variety of environmental stimuli, parental care and protection do not stop at birth. On the contrary, mammalian parents care for their newborn and preadult young for an extended period after birth. The duration and extent of postnatal care depend upon the length of time needed for the infant to acquire the ability to care for itself. The scope of postnatal parental care encompasses protection from predators, teaching certain skills necessary for survival, and seeing to nutritional needs. Mammals are distinguished from all other animals by suckling the infant from special milk-producing glands in the mother's pectoral region called mammary glands. It is the presence of mammary glands from which the term *mammal* is derived.

Of all infant mammals the human child requires the longest period of parental care, usually as long as 15 years or perhaps even 20. Unlike the newborn of other mammalian species, the newborn human lacks all but the most rudimentary degree of neuromuscular coordination. Soon after birth, for example, a young horse is able to stand, which it must do to nurse, and not long after that it is able to run, which it must do in order to stay with its mother and the herd. In contrast to the young horse, the human infant is virtually helpless in the several months after birth.

It cannot hold its own head erect until it is about three months old, cannot stand until the age of about 12 months, and usually cannot walk until it is well over a year old.

Since the child's survival abilities are severely limited, it is totally dependent upon adult caretakers for survival until it has acquired the skills and coordination to live successfully on its own. The adult caretakers, most often the parents, provide the child with an environment which promotes its physical, cognitive, and affective development. They see to the child's nutritional needs, they teach appropriate behavior, and they attend to the child's emotional needs. It is interesting to note that the newborn and the infant human child possess a limited behavioral repertoire by which the child specifically adapts to an environment of adult caretaking. Among these behaviors are sucking, crying, grasping, and smiling—each an innate ability that elicits a response from an adult which satisfies a particular need.

The extensive period of postnatal care is related to the time required for the brain to grow and for the child to achieve the coordination to stand, walk, and talk. At birth the child's head volume is less than one third the eventual adult size and less than one fourth the eventual adult weight. The complete anatomical and functional development of the human brain takes several years (Figure 1–5). The greatest period of brain growth occurs during the first year of life when the brain more than doubles in volume and weight and attains nearly 80 percent of its adult size. During this time the child begins to acquire the abilities of coordinated movement and speech, which are critical to the unfolding of more complex behavior later in life, such as abstract thought, reason, and imagination. It is these mental capabilities which distinguish man from other animals and which have led to man's successful adaptation to life on earth.

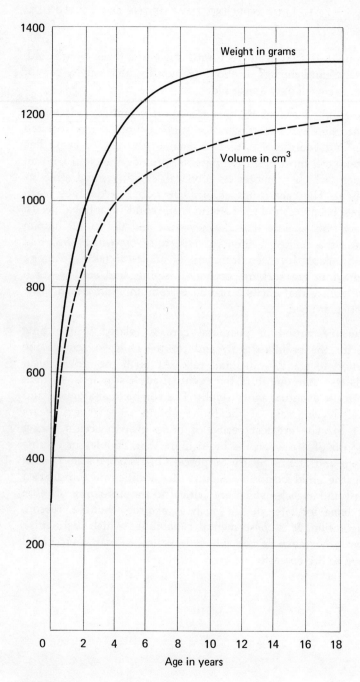

FIGURE 1-5
Growth of the human brain.

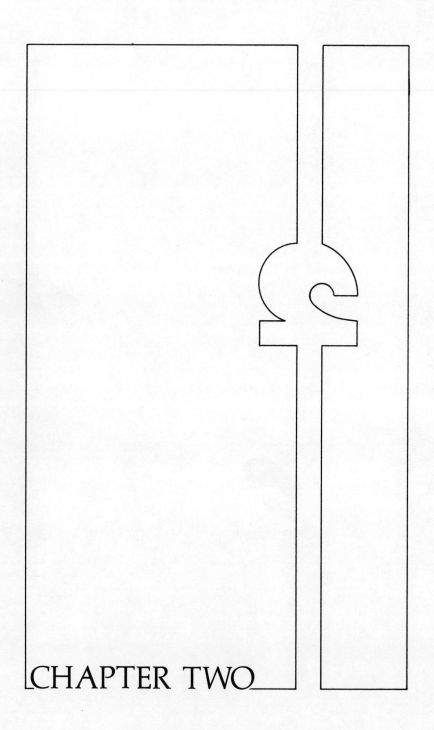

CHAPTER TWO

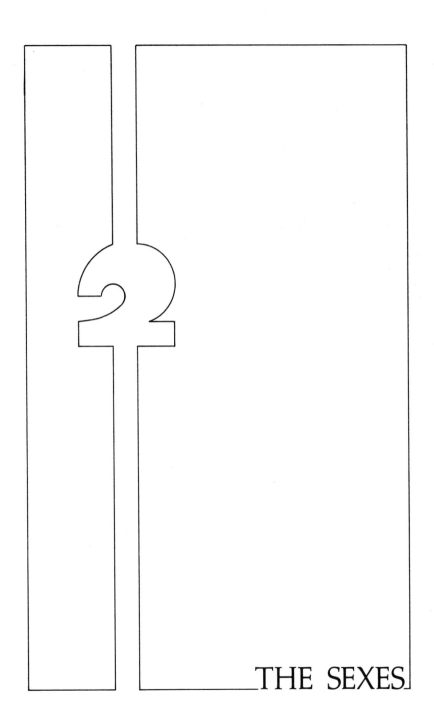

2

THE SEXES

One of the most obvious aspects of human reproduction is that it involves the participation of two people—a man and a woman—whose anatomy, physiology, and behavior are sexually distinct. The organs of the reproductive system are characteristically male or female. The size, shape, and stature of the body are characteristically male or female. All of these sexual characteristics are woven into a person's personality and create a sense of maleness or femaleness that affects one's self-concept and interactions with other people.

THE MALE REPRODUCTIVE SYSTEM

The male reproductive system consists of the pair of testes in which sperm and sex hormones are produced, the genital duct system through which sperm are transported from their site of production in the testes to the outside, a glandular system that produces seminal plasma, and the penis, the male organ of copulation (Figure 2–1).

THE TESTES

The *testes* are oval-shaped organs measuring about 3 cm in length and 2 cm in width. They are sometimes described as having the size and shape of eggs. The testes are located in a saclike structure that is attached to the lower, front portion of the pelvis (Figure 2–2). This structure is called the *scrotum*. Each of the testes is suspended in the scrotum at the end of a spermatic cord, a fibrous structure that contains nerves, blood vessels, a sperm duct called the *vas deferens*, and a thin muscle called the cremaster. The cremaster surrounds the testis, and its function is to raise the testis closer to the body in response to such stimuli as cold, fear, anger, and sexual stimulation. Usually the left testis hangs in the scrotum somewhat lower than the right testis.

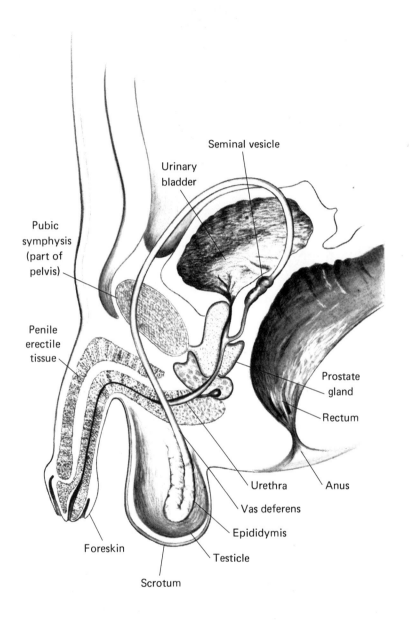

FIGURE 2-1
The male reproductive system.

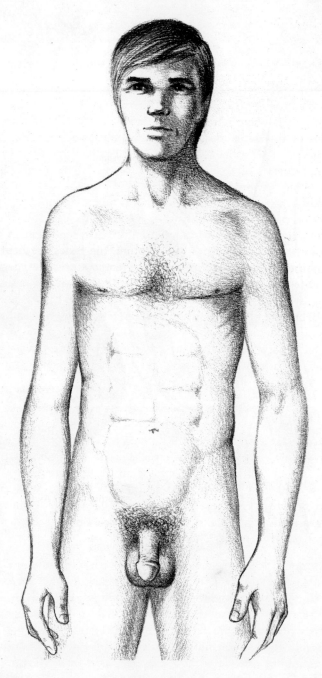

FIGURE 2-2
The testes are situated outside the body in the scrotum.

In the human fetus the testes develop inside the body, but shortly before birth they descend into the scrotum where they remain for life.

The descent of the testes from an internal location to one outside the body in the scrotum occurs in most mammalian species, and the time of the testes' descent is often correlated with the breeding season of the particular species. For example, the testes of bats and some species of rodent descend into the scrotum only during the breeding season and return to their original position inside the body when the breeding season is over. In humans, where there is no particular breeding season, the testes descend into the scrotum approximately two months before birth and remain there throughout life. While inside the scrotum, the testes are kept at a temperature below the normal body temperature, the decrease being three to five degrees in humans and as much as seven degrees in other animals. It has been found that sperm development is prevented at the internal body temperature, and thus it appears that the descent of the testes into the scrotum has evolved as an aid to sperm production, occurring at breeding seasons in animals which are seasonal breeders, and being a permanent condition in continuously breeding species like man.

Each testis is subdivided by connective tissue membranes into several hundred small lobules, and each of these lobules contains one or several coiled ducts called *seminiferous tubules* (Figure 2–3). It is in the lining of the seminiferous tubules that sperm are produced. The seminiferous tubules have an average diameter of 200 microns, but their overall uncoiled length is over 200 meters (Bloom & Fawcett, 1968). Interspersed among the seminiferous tubules are clusters of cells, called interstitial cells, which synthesize and release steroid sex hormones.

Sex hormones are biochemical agents which primarily influence the structure and function of the sex organs and the appearance of specific sexual characteristics; sex hormones also influence certain forms of behavior. The hormones which tend to produce male-type physical characteristics and behaviors are referred to as *androgens*, whereas the hormones which are capable of inducing many feminine characteristics are the *estrogens* (Figure 2–4)

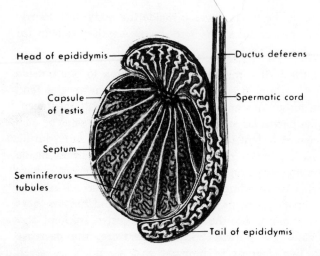

FIGURE 2-3
Seminiferous tubules in the testis. From C. Dienhart, *Basic Human Anatomy and Physiology* (Philadelphia: Saunders, 1973). Reprinted by permission.

(Table 2–1). An additional class of female hormones are the *progestogens*. These agents prepare the uterus to accept a fetus and are also necessary for the maintenance of a successful pregnancy. Androgens, estrogens, and progestogens are produced by both sexes. As one might expect, androgens are produced in greater amounts in males than females, and estrogens and progestogens are produced in greater amounts in females than males.

MALE GENITAL DUCTS

To provide an exit pathway for the sperm produced in the testes, there is a connected series of ducts which lead from the seminiferous tubules to the urethra of the penis, and hence outside the body (Figure 2–5). The first group of these sperm ducts are in the testis itself. They are the ductules comprising the *rete testis*—an interlacing network of short ducts into which the sperm from the

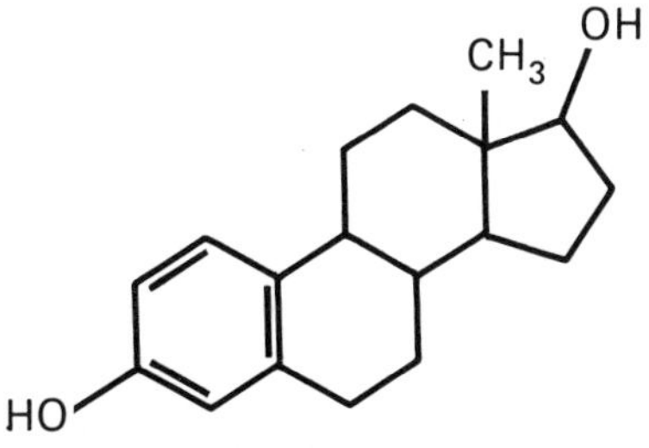

Estrogen (17 B Estradial)

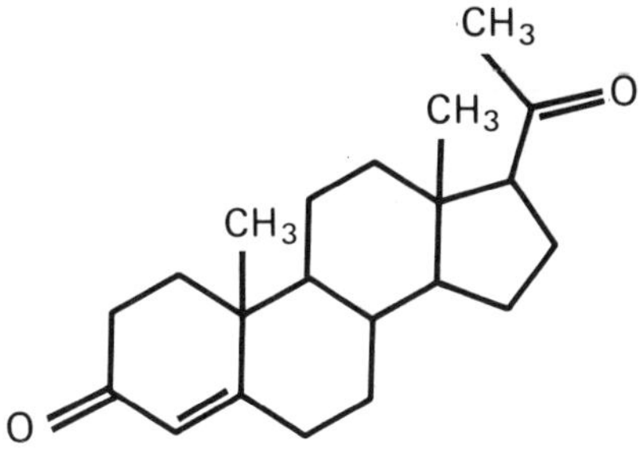

Progesterone

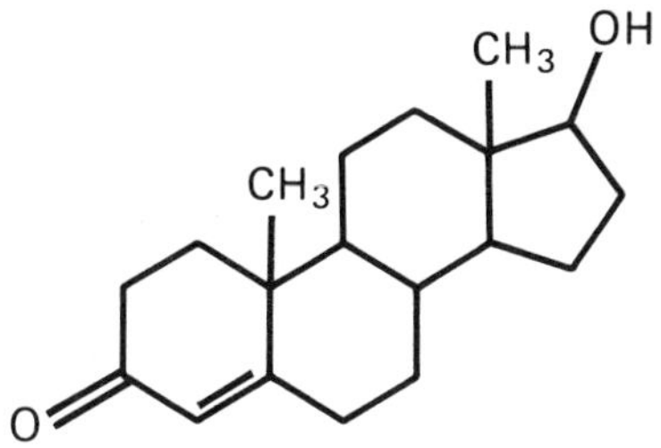

Androgen (Testosterone)

FIGURE 2-4
Chemical structures of sex steroid hormones.

TABLE 2.1
FUNCTIONS OF SEX STEROID HORMONES

ESTROGENS

Ovary
Increase sensitivity of granulosa cells to FSH and LH
Increase mitotic activity in germinal epithelium

Uterine Tubes
Increase motility
Increase secretion

Uterus
Proliferation of blood vessels and glands in endometrium
Increase size of muscle cells
Production of cervical fluid

Vagina
Stimulate growth and changes in vaginal cells
Maintenance of vaginal secretions

Breasts
Growth and development of nipple, areola, ducts

Secondary Sex Characteristics
Feminine pattern of hair growth
Feminine pattern of fat distribution

PROGESTOGENS

Uterine Tubes
Decrease motility of uterine tubes

Uterus
Increase secretory activity of endometrium
Decrease contractility of myometrium
Changes in viscocity of cervical fluid

Vagina
Changes in vaginal epithelium

ANDROGENS

Secondary Sex Characteristics
Male pattern of hair growth: beard, chest, abdomen, baldness
Increase muscle mass
Growth of larynx

Increase oil production in sebaceous glands

Genitalia
Promote growth and function of penis, scrotum, prostate, seminal vesicles
Support sperm production
Affect composition of seminal fluid

Libido
Promote sex drive

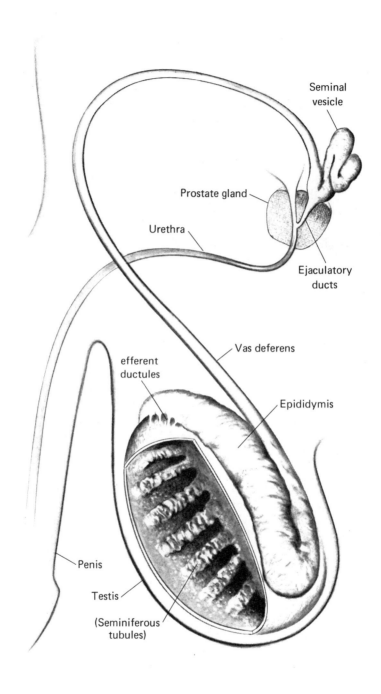

Seminal
vesicle

Prostate gland

Urethra

Ejaculatory
ducts

Vas deferens

efferent
ductules

Epididymis

Penis

Testis

(Seminiferous
tubules)

FIGURE 2-5
Male genital ducts.

many seminiferous tubules collect. The tubules of the rete testis are joined to 10 to 15 short, straight ducts referred to as *efferent ductules*. These ducts transport the sperm from the rete testis to a duct lying on the back portion of the testis called the *epididymis*.

The epididymis is a highly coiled duct that is encased in a connective tissue covering. The duct itself is about 5 meters long, but coiled as it is, the actual length of the entire organ is only about 3 or 4 cm. As the sperm mature in the testes they are transported to each adjacent epididymis, where they are stored until ejaculation. When the male ejaculates, the smooth muscle that makes up part of the wall of the epididymis contracts, setting up propulsive forces which move the sperm out of the epididymis.

After they leave the epididymis, the sperm enter and are subsequently propelled along a duct called the *vas deferens*. There are two such ducts, each leading within a spermatic cord from an epididymis toward the lower part of the bladder. There each vas connects to a short, straight duct about 2 cm long called an *ejaculatory duct*. Each ejaculatory duct has a separate opening into the urethra, so the sperm from each testis are joined into one mass before leaving the male's body through the urethra of the penis.

On the journey from the seminiferous tubules of the testes to the penis, the sperm become mixed with the milky white seminal plasma, which makes up the bulk of the total ejaculate. The components of seminal plasma are produced by three glands closely associated with the sperm duct system: the *seminal vesicles*, a pair of saccular glands which are outpocketings of the vas deferens; the *prostate gland*, which surrounds the urethra near its origin at the bladder and which has 16 to 32 short ducts that open into the urethra; the *bulbourethral glands*, a pair of fluid-producing glands, each about the size of a pea and having ducts that enter into the urethra. The final total ejaculate, then, is made up of sperm from the seminiferous tubules and seminal plasma from the seminal vesicles, prostate, and bulbourethral glands. The volume of an average ejaculate is approximately 4 cubic centimeters (cc). Over 99 percent of this volume is contributed by the seminal plasma whereas the remaining 1 percent is composed of 300 million to 500 million sperm.

THE PENIS

The penis is the male organ of copulation. It is involved in the sexual stimulation of both sex partners during sexual intercourse and in the deposition of sperm in the female vagina.

The males of most mammalian species, such as bears, dogs, and seals, have a bone which runs the length of the penis, thereby creating a stiff structure which can be inserted easily into the vagina. In humans, however, there is no penile bone, as the penis is composed primarily of erectile tissue. Normally the penis is limp and incapable of penetrating the vagina. When a man becomes sexually excited, however, the blood vessels that carry blood into the penis dilate and the blood flow into the erectile tissue of the penis increases, causing the penis to become hard and erect, thus making intromission possible (Figure 2–6). In the flaccid state, the penis is approximately 9 cm long and about 3 cm in diameter. When the penis becomes erect, it lengthens an additional 8 cm, and its diameter increases to about 4 cm (Masters and Johnson, 1966). There is no relationship between the size of the penis, either flaccid or erect, and a man's general body build.

The body of the penis is composed of three cylindrical structures, two *corpora cavernosa* and a single *corpus spongiosum* (Figure 2–7). These are the erectile components of the penis. The two corpora cavernosa lie next to one another and make up the top or dorsal side of the penis. The corpus spongiosum lies underneath the corpora cavernosa; it contains the urethra through which the man urinates and ejaculates. When the male ejaculates, the portion of the urethra near the bladder is pinched off so only sperm can pass through the penis. This prevents the simultaneous emission of both urine and semen and also prevents the movement of sperm into the bladder instead of through the penis.

At the time of birth, the penis has a fold of skin covering the tip; this fold is called the *foreskin* or prepuce. Since ancient times, the Jewish people have by custom surgically removed the foreskin from the penis of newborn males within a few days after birth. This operation, called circumcision, is now common practice in many United States hospitals regardless of the religion or cultural heritage of the child.

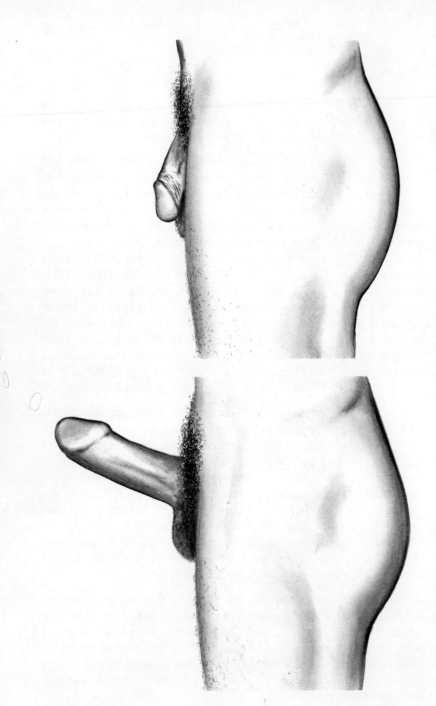

FIGURE 2-6
Erection of the penis.

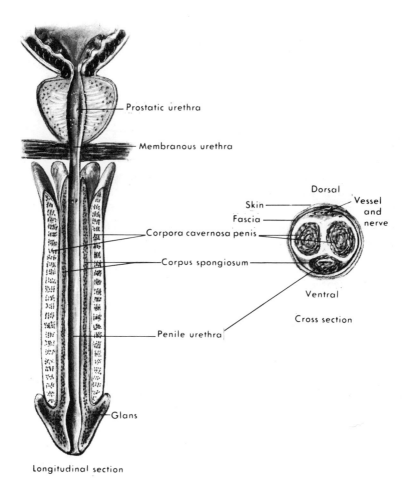

Longitudinal section

FIGURE 2-7
Anatomy of the penis. From C. Dienhart, *Basic Human Anatomy and Physiology* (Philadelphia: Saunders, 1973). Reprinted by permission.

THE FEMALE
REPRODUCTIVE
SYSTEM

The female reproductive system consists of the pair of ovaries in which ova and sex hormones are produced, the pair of uterine

27

tubes where fertilization takes place, a uterus where the fertilized ovum develops into a fetus, and a vagina through which the fetus emerges from the mother's body at birth (Figure 2–8). The vagina is also the woman's copulatory organ, and associated with the vagina are several sexually sensitive genital organs.

THE OVARIES

The ovaries of the human female are slightly flattened oval-shaped organs about 3 cm long, 2 cm wide, and 1 cm thick. They are located in the pelvic cavity where they lie separated from each other by the uterus and the pair of uterine tubes (Figure 2–9).

The ova are found near the surface of the ovary, surrounded by clusters of nutrient and hormone-secreting cells. Each ovum and its contingent of encircling cells is called an *ovarian follicle*. At birth, the number of ovarian follicles present in both ovaries ranges between 500,000 and 700,000. None of the ova in these follicles is ready for fertilization, however. They must first undergo a maturation process which does not begin until a female reaches puberty. At that time, and for the next three or four decades of life, an ovum capable of taking part in fertilization is released from its follicle approximately every 28 days. The sex hormones secreted by the ovaries are principally estrogen and progesterone.

UTERINE TUBES

Situated between each ovary and the uterus is a *uterine* or *fallopian tube*, sometimes called the oviduct. Each of the uterine tubes is about 10 cm long with a diameter of about 0.5 cm. The end of the uterine tube nearest the ovary opens into the abdominal cavity. The uterine end of the tube is connected to the uterus, such that the cavity of the uterine tube is continuous with the cavity of the uterus (Figure 2–10).

The uterine tubes are very important structures in human reproduction, for it is within the tubes that fertilization takes place. Sperm which are deposited in the vagina during sexual inter-

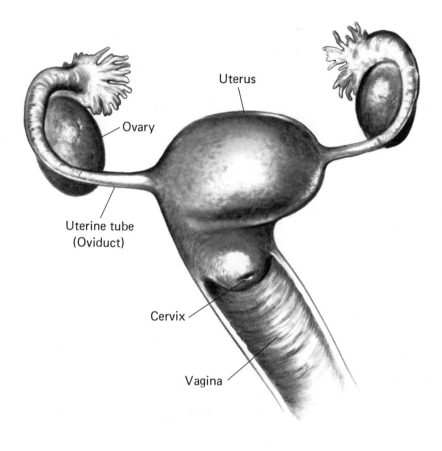

FIGURE 2-8
Female reproductive system.

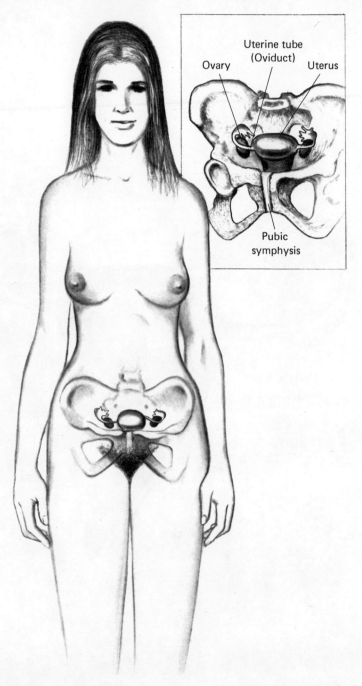

FIGURE 2-9
Position of female reproductive organs in the pelvic cavity.

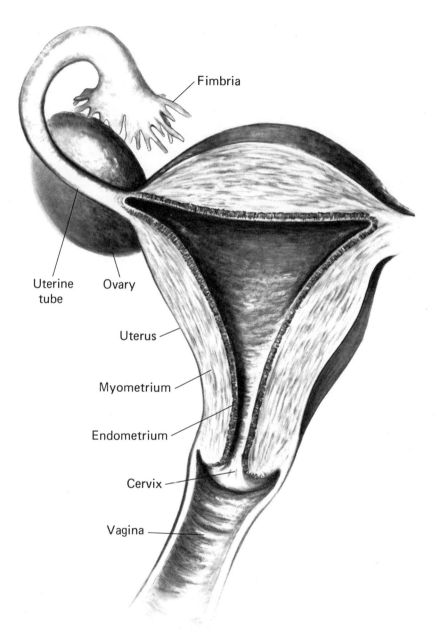

FIGURE 2-10
Cross section of the uterus, uterine tubes, and ovary.

course migrate through the cervix and body of the uterus and into the tubes. An ovum released from the ovary enters the open end of the tube so it can rendezvous with a sperm.

Because the uterine tube and the ovary are not completely connected (although there is a small projection from the ovarian end of the tube which is often applied directly to the surface of the ovary), ovulation releases ova into the abdominal cavity. In order for fertilization to occur inside the tube, the ovum must enter the open end of the uterine tube. Capture of the ovum after it is released from the ovary is apparently facilitated by tentaclelike projections, called *fimbriae*, located at the ovarian end of the tubes and also movements of the tubes themselves which bring the open, fimbriated ends of the tubes close to the ovary.

After the ovum has entered the tube, and after it has been fertilized, the tubes facilitate the transport of the fertilized ovum to the uterus where subsequent development of the fetus takes place. The inner lining of the tubes contains cells which have microscopic hairlike structures called cilia projecting from their surface into the cavity of the tube. The cilia beat in the direction of the uterus and act like many thousands of fingers which move the fertilized ovum toward the uterus. In addition to the beat of the cilia, transport of the fertilized ovum to the uterus is aided by contractions of the tube itself.

THE UTERUS
AND VAGINA

The *uterus* of an adult woman is a hollow, somewhat pear-shaped organ situated in the pelvic cavity in the midline of the body between the urinary bladder and the rectum (Figure 2–11). At the upper, rounded portion of the uterus are attached the two uterine tubes, one on each side. The lower narrow end of the uterus extends into the vagina. This portion of the uterus is called the *cervix* (cervix = neck). The normal, nonpregnant uterus is about the size of a woman's closed fist—approximately 7 cm long and 5 cm wide at the upper end. The width of the cervix is about 3 cm. During pregnancy the upper portion of the uterus expands considerably in order to accommodate the growing fetus, the placenta,

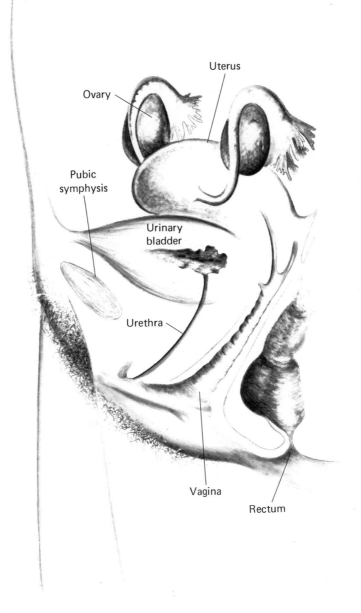

Ovary

Uterus

Pubic
symphysis

Urinary
bladder

Urethra

Vagina

Rectum

FIGURE 2-11
Cross section of female pelvic organs.

the fetal membranes, and amniotic fluid. The cervix, being composed of mostly fibrous tissues, does not expand during pregnancy. It maintains its relative stiffness in order to retain the uterine contents.

The uterus is composed of three major tissue layers. The innermost layer which lines the uterine cavity is called the *endometrium*. The endometrium is supplied with many blood vessels and contains secretory cells. Adjacent to the endometrium is a muscular layer called the *myometrium*. The smooth muscle cells of the myometrium provide the strong propulsive forces necessary to expel the fetus at birth. The outermost layer of the uterus is composed of fibrous connective tissue which makes up part of the ligamentous structures that support the uterus in the pelvic cavity and connect it to the body wall.

The *vagina* is a cylindrical, thin-walled muscular tube with one end joined to the uterine cervix and the other end open to the outside. The vagina is between 8 and 10 cm long, and it extends into the body at an upward angle of approximately 45 degrees. Normally the vaginal canal is only a potential space, for the walls of the vagina usually lie very close together. The vaginal canal is quite distensible, however, and can readily expand to receive the penis during sexual intercourse or to allow passage of a baby at birth.

The vagina of most newborn girls has a skinlike piece of tissue at the entrance of the vagina called the *hymen*. Hymens vary in size and can cover the entire opening, or hardly be large enough to cover it at all; in some women the hymen may be completely absent from birth.

The region of a woman's body where the vagina opens to the outside is referred to as the vaginal vestibule. The vaginal vestibule is located in the lower front portion of the pelvis between the woman's legs. In addition to the vagina, the female urethra, through which the woman urinates, also opens into the vaginal vestibule about 1 cm above the vaginal opening. The opening of the urethra is called the urethral meatus. In close association with the vestibule are the female external genitalia: the *mons pubis*, the *labia majora*, the *labia minora*, and the *clitoris* (Figure 2–12). The mons pubis is an elevation of subcutaneous fatty tissue

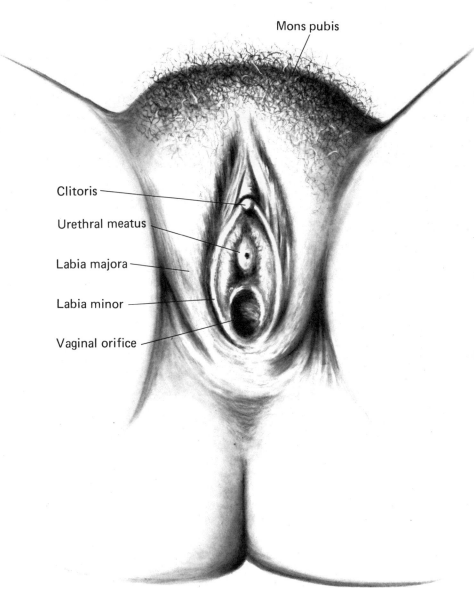

Mons pubis

Clitoris

Urethral meatus

Labia majora

Labia minor

Vaginal orifice

FIGURE 2-12
Female external genitalia.

located above the vestibule and in the adult woman is covered with pubic hair. The labia majora protrude from the sides of the vestibule and extend toward the midline, tending to cover the vestibule. The labia minora are smaller folds which are covered by the labia majora. And situated between the labia minora about 2 cm above the urethral opening is the clitoris. The clitoris is similar in structure to the male penis in that it is composed of erectile tissue, but it is a smaller organ than the penis measuring about 2 cm in length and about 1 cm in diameter, and although it engorges with blood when a woman becomes sexually excited, it does not enlarge as greatly as does the penis. However, like the penis, the clitoris is supplied with many sensory nerves which make it an extremely sensitive organ.

EMBRYONIC DEVELOPMENT OF SEX ORGANS

Both the testes and the ovaries form during the fifth week of development from a pair of thickenings in the posterior wall of the embryonic abdominal cavity (Figure 2–13). These thickenings are called the *genital ridges*, and in their earliest stages of development they are anatomically similar in both male and female embryos. If the sex chromosomes of the embryo are the XY pair of a male, then the genital ridges differentiate into the testes. If, on the other hand, the sex chromosomes are the XX pair of a female, then the genital ridges differentiate into the ovaries.

The germ cells, the sperm and ova, do not develop from the tissue comprising the genital ridges, as we might expect. Instead, the primordial germ cells originate in a nongonadal embryonic structure called the yolk sac, and they become part of the gonads by migrating from the yolk sac to the genital ridges. The migration of the primordial germ cells begins about the fourth week of development and is completed a little over a week later.

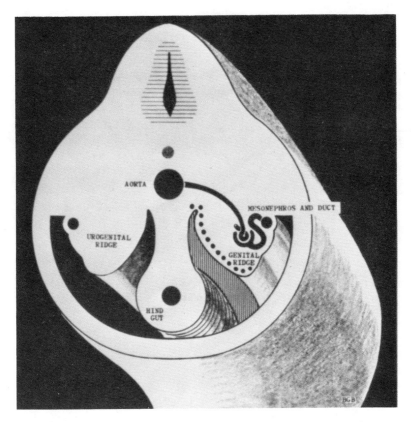

FIGURE 2-13
Cross section of 4-week-old embryo. Primordial germ cells (black dots) migrate from the region of the hindgut to the genital ridges. From J. P. Greenhill, *Obstetrics*, 13th ed. (Philadelphia: Saunders, 1965). Reprinted by permission.

The internal genitalia in both male and female embryos develop from one or the other of two sets of paired undifferentiated genital duct systems that are present in the fetus by the sixth week of embryonic life. These two duct systems are called the mesonephric ducts and the paramesonephric ducts; they extend from the region of the fetal kidney in the abdominal cavity into the pelvic cavity (Figure 2–14). In a normal male embryo at about eight weeks of

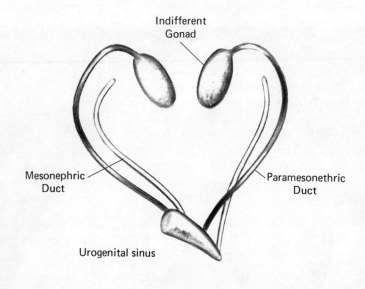

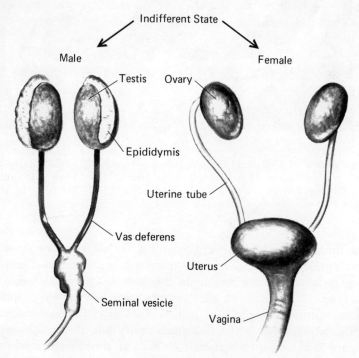

FIGURE 2-14
Fate of mesonephric and paramesonephric ducts.

development, an "inductor substance" (or substances) is elaborated from the fetal testis which diffuses into the region of the mesonephric and paramesonephric ducts on the same side of the body and induces the differentiation of the male internal genitalia on that side—the epididymis, vas deferens, the seminal vesicle, and the ejaculatory duct—and also the regression of the paramesonephric duct, except for some minor remnants. In the female embryo, such an inductor substance is not emitted, in which case the mesonephric ducts degenerate and the paramesonephric ducts differentiate into the female internal genitalia. The upper ends of the two paramesonephric ducts become the uterine tubes and the lower ends fuse to become the uterus and the upper four fifths of the vagina.

As in the case with the development of the gonads and the internal genital ducts, the external genitalia develop from anatomical structures that are at first sexually indistinct in both male and female embryos. In the five-week-old embryo, the precursors of the external genitalia in both sexes consist of a genital tubercle, a pair of genital folds, and a pair of genital swellings (Figure 2–15). In the male, the genital tubercle develops into the penis whereas in the female it develops into the clitoris. The genital folds differentiate into the penile urethra in the male or the labia minora in the female. And the genital swellings fuse to become the scrotum in the male, or remain separated as the labia majora in the female.

The differentiation of the genital tubercle, genital folds, and genital swellings into the male external genitalia appears to be under the control of androgenic compounds elaborated by the fetal testis, and without the presence of these androgenic compounds, embryos develop the external genitalia of females regardless of the genetic sex. Experiments on laboratory animals have demonstrated this effect quite well. If genetic male embryos are castrated before the differentiation of their external genitalia, thus removing a major source of fetal androgens, they develop the external genital organs of a female. Conversely, if exogenous testosterone is given to fetal genetic females, they are born with the genitalia of males, having a penis and scrotum instead of clitoris and vaginal labia. Thus it appears that all embryos will develop the external genitalia of females unless some type of androgen is present to induce the masculine form.

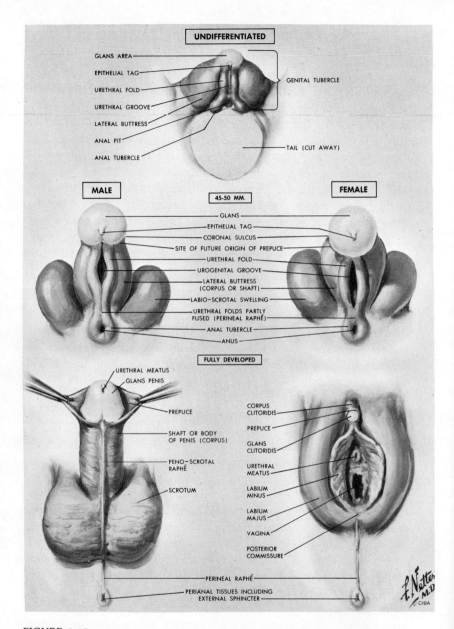

FIGURE 2-15

Homologues of external male and female genitalia; development from undifferentiated to differentiated stage. © Copyright 1965 by CIBA Pharmaceutical Company, Division of CIBA-Geigy Corp. Reproduced with permission from the CIBA Collection of Medical Illustrations by Frank H. Netter, M.D. All rights reserved.

SECONDARY SEX
CHARACTERISTICS

There are a number of anatomical differences between men and women in addition to the aforementioned differences in the principal sexual organs (Figure 2–16). Because these sexually distinct physical attributes are not involved in the production of germ cells or their eventual union at fertilization, they are referred to as secondary sex characteristics. Some examples of feminine secondary sex characteristics are the presence of breasts, a relatively wide pelvis and the distribution of subcutaneous body fat on the hips, buttocks, thighs, and calves, all of which gives the average female body its characteristic contoured appearance. Male secondary sex characteristics include broad shoulders and slim hips, and a greater proportion of muscle in relation to body fat. Men also have a larger larynx so their voices tend to be low. Men tend to have more hair on their legs, arms, and torso than women, and of the two sexes only men normally grow beards. Both sexes normally grow hair under their arms (axillary hair) and in the genital region (pubic hair).

The secondary sex characteristics begin to appear in adolescence during a phase of life known as puberty. *Puberty* is the time of life when a person's body undergoes the physical changes necessary to become capable of reproduction. The onset of puberty is triggered by the increased production of pituitary gonadotropic hormones, follicle stimulating hormone (FSH) and luteinizing hormone (LH), which in turn stimulate the growth of the gonads and the production of steroid sex hormones. In adolescent males the testes thus begin to secrete large amounts of testosterone, and in adolescent females the ovaries make large amounts of estrogen, principally estradiol. These hormones, along with other steroid hormones secreted by the adrenal cortex, induce the formation of the secondary sex characteristics, and they also stimulate the further growth and the functional maturation of the genital organs.

In girls puberty usually begins between the ages of 10½ and 12, and the period of change normally lasts about three years. Very often the beginning of breast development is the first noticeable

41

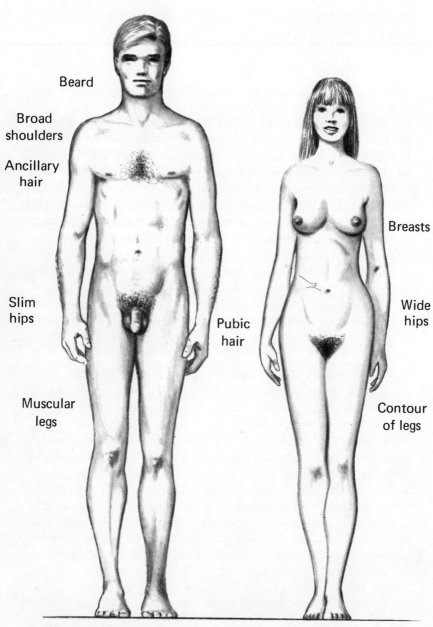

FIGURE 2-16
Secondary sex characteristics.

sign of puberty, although the appearance of pubic hair may sometimes come before breast growth. Soon after puberty has begun, the uterus and vagina begin to grow. In the ensuing years the breasts continue to develop; the hips become wide in comparison to the waist; subcutaneous fat accumulates on the hips, thighs, and buttocks; and perhaps the most important of all, the girl experiences her first menstrual period, known as the *menarche*.

Puberty begins in boys between the ages of 12½ and 14. This is about two years later than the beginning of puberty in girls. The duration of puberty in boys is longer than the period of puberty in girls, however, lasting on the average about five years. Sometimes some of the physical changes in a male are not complete until he has reached his early twenties.

The first sign of puberty in a male is growth of the testes and scrotum. Pubic hair also begin to appear at this time. About a year after the onset of testicular growth, the penis begins to grow, the shoulders broaden, the larynx enlarges, and facial hair becomes prominent. Also at this time the seminal vesicles and prostate begin to grow, soon becoming functional and producing seminal fluid. This allows the young man to experience ejaculation for the first time in his life.

SEXUAL BEHAVIOR

In virtually all human societies certain behavioral characteristics are associated with maleness and other behavioral characteristics with femaleness. The specifics of sex-typed behavior very often differ in detail from society to society and from time to time in any given society. For example, in some societies only men perform agricultural tasks whereas in others only women do. And in most Western cultures including ours, men are expected to be the initiators of sexual activity, but in several other societies the women initiate sexual encounters (Ford & Beach, 1953).

In American society the generally accepted model of masculine behavior is that a man competes for economic resources, sharing what he has acquired with a chosen mate and any children they have. Men are also expected to defend themselves, their families, and the society with acts of physical violence. To fulfill these expectations and other duties of their sex role, men are expected to be more aggressive, logical, brave, independent, and unemotional than women.

The sex role for women generally restricts them to domestic duties. The cultural expectation is that women are supposed to marry, see to the physical, emotional, and sexual needs of outgoing and hardworking husbands, and care for the home and children. To fulfill this role women are expected to be more emotional, non-aggressive, dependent, and seductive than men.

It has been suggested that the stereotypic American sex roles—the male as protector and provider and the female as primary child caretaker and homemaker—are vestiges of a division of labor based on sex that might have existed in the first human groups. Anthropological theory suggests that the early hominids were nomadic hunters that roamed the plains of Africa looking for food. By virtue of their strength and agility, the males of these groups fought and hunted, whereas the females, their mobility hindered by the needs of small children to be breast-fed and cared for, probably had to depend on the fighting and hunting skills of a male to help feed and protect them and their children.

While such sex-specific behavior may have been necessary for the survival of early humans, the male role as provider and female role as home and child caretaker must be viewed as adaptive behaviors aiding the survival of a particular human group in a given ecological time and place. Although the task of child rearing has traditionally befallen women, this need not be the case in present-day technologically advanced countries. Modern pediatric practices allow parents to leave the care of children to professionals. It is even possible for the traditional sex roles to become reversed. In some families the wife assumes the role of provider by going out to work and the husband remains at home to look after the needs of children and do housework.

It appears that sex-specific behavior is predominantly learned in childhood based largely upon a child's knowledge of its own sex and the subsequent emulation of sex-specific behavior observed in model adults, most often the parents or other authority figures.

These adults influence the development of the child's sex-specific behavior by rewarding what they consider to be proper behavior and by punishing what is considered to be improper behavior. Children of both sexes are exposed to a variety of rules which dictate what little boys should or should not do and what little girls should and should not do. Children as young as three years old can cite a long list of behavior expected of them as members of their sex as well as behavior characteristic of the opposite sex.

Parents treat their children as members of one sex and not the other based on their knowledge of the child's anatomical sex, which they usually gain at birth from the appearance of the newborn child's external genitalia. Thus babies born with male external genitalia are assigned a masculine sex and are thereafter treated as boys. They come to identify as members of the male gender and grow up assimilating the behavioral characteristics expected of adult males. The analogous process occurs in babies born with female external genitalia. They are assigned the feminine gender, treated as girls in their young lives, and consequently assimilate the feminine sex-typed behavior expected of adult women.

Evidence to support the hypothesis that sex-specific behavior is learned comes from studies of children who were born with developmental abnormalities in which the appearance of the external genitalia at birth was ambiguous or even characteristic of the opposite sex (Hampson and Hampson, 1961). For example, some of the genetic male children in the study were born with the developmental abnormality called testicular feminization or the androgen insensitivity syndrome. In this instance the fetal tissues are unresponsive to androgen and hence the genitalia do not develop in the normal pattern. Instead, the external genitalia appear feminine: the penis is small and resembles a clitoris; the scrotum is not fused and therefore resembles the major labia; and there may be a short vagina. Because the child is a genetic male he has testes, but they remain undescended in the abdominal cavity.

Since the true genetic sex of these children born with androgen insensitivity syndrome was not determined at birth, they were assigned the sex of females and raised by their parents as girls. The children grew up identifying as females and displayed behavioral characteristics of women. Frequently the truth about the condition was not discovered until adolescence when the young girls failed to begin menstruating. By this time, it was impossible to reverse the feminine identity, to make it correspond to the genetic male sex, and the young women continued their lives as females.

An analogous developmental defect which affects genetic females is called the adrenogenital syndrome. In this instance a genetic female fetus becomes "masculinized" because of a metabolic defect which causes a hypersecretion of androgen from the fetal adrenal glands. The excessive amounts of androgen override the feminine developmental process and produce masculine appearing genitalia. The clitoris of the newborn child is often enlarged to the degree that it resembles the penis of a newborn male child, and the labia majora can fuse to form what appears to be a scrotal sac. Individuals born with adrenogenital syndrome may be assigned the male sex, thereafter reared as boys, and adopt masculine sexual identities and sex-specific behavior.

From experiments on laboratory animals it appears that the sexual behavior of both males and females can be influenced by gonadal sex hormones (Money and Ehrhardt, 1972). One generalization to emerge from the research, for example, is that androgens produce characteristically male-type behavior in test animals (aggression, dominance, mounting, pelvic thrusting), and that estrogen and progesterone produce feminine behavior (docility, lordosis, maternal behavior). This and other experimental work have invited the hypothesis that some aspects of human behavior are influenced by sex hormones. For example, there is evidence to suggest that androgens maintain the sex drive (libido) in both sexes (see Chapter 3). There is also some evidence to indicate that the low blood levels of estrogen and progesterone that occur at the time of menstruation and at the end of pregnancy are related to the severe changes in mood experienced by many women at these times, namely, "premenstrual syndrome" and "postpartum blues" (Dalton, 1964).

Another hypothesis under investigation is that hormones in fetal life affect brain development in a masculine or feminine way. Laboratory experiments with monkeys suggest that the presence in fetal life of significant amounts of androgen induces the postnatal display of masculine behavior (play initiation, rough and tumble play, chasing play).

That androgen present in fetal life might affect humans as it does monkeys is suggested by behavioral observations of female children with the adrenogenital syndrome, but who were sex-assigned correctly at birth in concordance with their genetic sex (XX = female), rather than assigned the sex corresponding to the appearance of their external genitalia (male). Since they were assigned the feminine gender, they were raised as females and adopted a feminine identity. Nevertheless, observations of these girls revealed a preponderance of certain behavior considered masculine. Most of these girls, for example, were considered "tomboys." They had high levels of energy which they chose to expend in vigorous outdoor games normally played by boys. In dress, these girls preferred to wear pants instead of dresses. And although they were not violently aggressive, they did tend to be competitive and dominant. These observations are taken to suggest that even though learning is the overriding determinant in the development of sex-specific behavior, it is still possible that hormones have some organizing effect on sexual behavior.

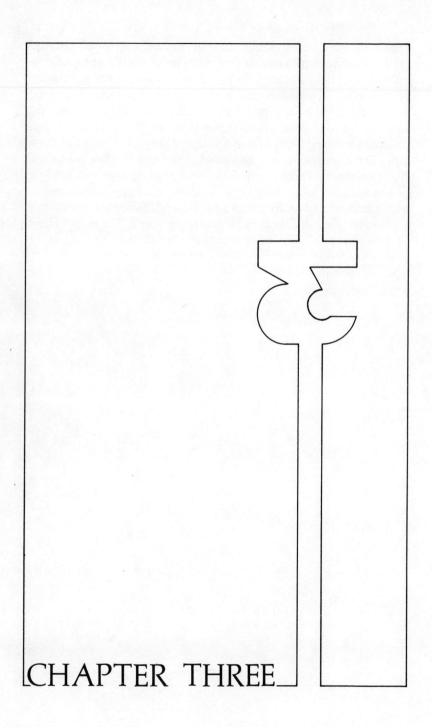

CHAPTER THREE

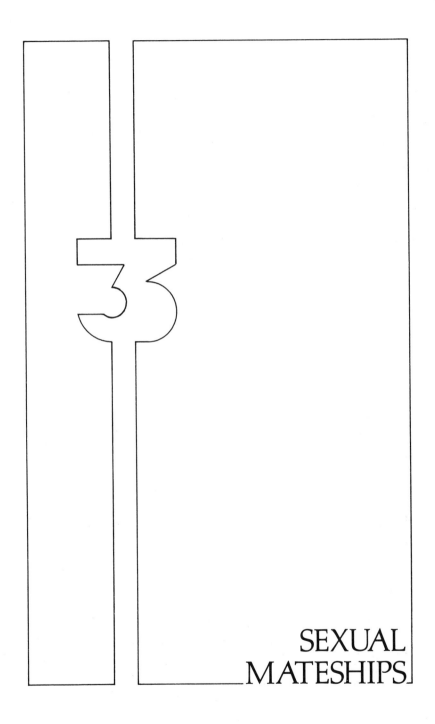

3

SEXUAL MATESHIPS

In many animal species, sexual behavior and the physical ability to mate are manifest only at times corresponding to the production of reproductively capable gametes. For example, in seasonally breeding animals, males and females display sexual behavior and become sexually active only during the breeding season when mature sperm and ova are being produced. At other times of the year sexual behavior and mating do not occur. In animals such as dogs, cats, and several primate species in which the adult male continuously produces mature sperm and the females produce ova only at certain intervals, the male always appears ready for sexual activity whereas the female is unwilling to copulate except at times in the fertility cycle when she is producing ova.

Human sexual activity differs from these examples in that women do not limit sexual activity to the time of ovum production. Like men, women are capable of sexual relations virtually all of the time, even though they are fertile for only a few days near the middle of the monthly menstrual cycle. As a consequence, one of the most distinctive aspects of human behavior is the degree to which sexual activity occurs without reference to the bearing of children. Human beings engage in sexual intercourse at a frequency far exceeding that needed to procreate the species. Indeed, a man and a woman who have established a monogamous reproductive mateship can produce a maximum of about thirty children, given that usually one ovum is fertilized at a time, that the gestation period of the human fetus is nine months, and that a woman normally takes a few weeks to recover from pregnancy before she is capable of becoming pregnant again. Contrast the 30 sexual contacts necessary to accomplish this maximum in human fecundity with the fact that the average American married couple engages in sexual intercourse between one and two times a week (Figure 3-1), which amounts to well over 1000 coital experiences in a lifetime (Kinsey et al., 1953).

One of the principal factors that motivates people to engage in frequent sexual relations is that men and women experience powerful and seemingly biologically generated urges which arouse in them the desire for sexual activity. These sexual urges are collectively referred to as the *sex drive*. They tend to create feelings of sexual tension and restlessness (sometimes referred to as being "horny") that are relieved when a person engages in sex.

A second factor which motivates people to take part in frequent

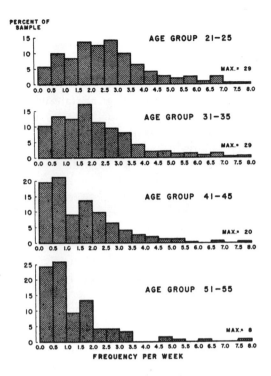

FIGURE 3-1
Frequency of sexual intercourse. From A. C. Kinsey, et al., *Sexual Behavior in the Human Female* (Philadelphia: Saunders, 1953). Reprinted by permission.

sexual relations is that sex can provide an opportunity to express one's deepest feelings, attitudes, and emotions. The most common feelings to be expressed sexually are love and affection. People expressing their love for one another sexually find that sex offers a means of interpersonal communication in much the same way that words and gestures (body-language) do. Indeed, sexual intercourse is sometimes described as "body conversation." Many people find that the expression of love through sex can give a feeling of spiritual transcendence, as if one's inner self has escaped the confines of the psyche and is freely interacting with that of the lover. There seems to be a consuming joining of spirits, just as there is joining of bodies. It is this simultaneous sharing of one's personality and body which makes sexual relations some of the most rewarding of life's experiences.

THE SEX DRIVE

The sex drive can be thought of as the psychological state which motivates people to seek out and engage in sexual activity. Like hunger and thirst, the sex drive is often considered to be one of the basic drive states that direct an individual's behavior toward a specific goal. Just as hunger and thirst motivate an individual to eat and drink, so the sex drive is thought to motivate an individual to participate in sexual activity. One major difference between the sex drive and the drives of hunger and thirst, however, is that sexual activity is not necessary to keep a person alive, whereas eating and drinking are. A person can go a lifetime without sexual experiences, as some people do for religious reasons, but no one can survive for very long without food and water. In spite of this difference, the sex drive is nevertheless considered one of the basic drive states because sexual activity is obligatory to the reproductive process and hence the survival of the species.

The character of the sex drive is often described as arousing in men and women feelings of sexual tension. These feelings characteristically involve an increased desire for physical sexual stimulation and also an increase in neuromuscular tension. Sexual tensions tend to be cumulative; they may begin as an almost unconscious interest in sex, but they may build to a consciously agitating level the longer sexual activity is postponed.

There are two general classes of stimuli which excite the sex drive in humans. One class consists of stimuli arising from outside the body (external stimuli) which are perceived by the sense organs (eyes, ears, nose, and so forth). The other class of stimuli arises from within the body itself (internal stimuli).

An example of an external sexually arousing stimulus is the sight of something or someone considered by the viewer as "sexy." The propensity of American men to become sexually aroused by visual stimuli has been chronicled by Kinsey (Kinsey et al., 1948, 1953), who reported that the sight of a woman's breasts, hips, legs, and buttocks tends to sexually excite most men, evoking erotic responses ranging from a general feeling of sexual arousal to penile erection and occasionally even ejaculation. Although women tend to become sexually aroused by the male physique, they are apparently not as stimulated by visual erotica as are men. This observation has been offered to explain why erotic movies, erotic magazines, and burlesque shows are directed principally at males.

The particular facets of the anatomy which are considered to be sexually appealing may differ from society to society. For example, in our culture a slim person is generally considered more sexually appealing than someone who is plump. However, in most other human societies the reverse is true with regard to the standard of the sexually appealing woman (Ford and Beach, 1953). Differences in the standard of sexual appeal can be found with regard to the size and shape of women's breasts, the porportions of the male physique, the color of the hair or skin.

Other sexually arousing stimuli include certain scents or odors (hence the wearing of pleasant smelling lotions, perfumes, and colognes), a provocative gesture, a particular kind of touch, or even a complex behavior such as a dance or a feat of strength or skill.

Little is known about the nature of internal stimuli that arouse sexual interest in people, but some observations have been made suggesting that the gonadal sex hormones influence the sex drive in humans. This is a reasonable proposition since the sexual activities of many nonhuman animals are influenced and often directly controlled by sex hormones. This is particularly true of seasonally breeding animals, who become sexually active only during a particular time of the year. Their sexual activity is triggered by an upsurge in the blood level of gonadal sex hormones occurring at the time of the breeding season. When these animals are out of their breeding seasons they can be experimentally induced to display their "in season" sexual behaviors by administering sex hormones to them; the androgens, primarily testosterone, can produce sexual activity in many male animals, and estrogen and progesterone, either singly or together, induce sexual behavior in female animals.

That testosterone or other potent male sex hormones influence the sex drive in human males is suggested by the observation that some men in whom the level of testosterone is low or absent often show a loss in sexual desire. These are men who have had their testes removed surgically (usually because of war injuries) or are men who have abnormally low amounts of testosterone production from intact but poorly functioning testes. Very often they experience a diminished sex drive even though the penis is fully capable of sexual performance. A loss in sex drive is also reported in many men who are given estrogens for prostate cancer. The effect of the estrogens is to lower the testicular output of testosterone which is designed to slow the growth of the hormone-dependent cancer cells.

The expectation that the sex drive in human females is influenced primarily by the sex hormones estrogen and progesterone, as it is in other animal females, is not borne out by observations of women who have had their ovaries removed (usually for the treatment of breast cancer). This operation significantly reduces a woman's levels of estrogen and progesterone by removing their primary source. Contrary to what is expected, many of the women who undergo the ovariectomy operation report that their sexual desires are unimpaired, and some even report an enhanced interest in sex because the fear of pregnancy is removed. However, in other surgical techniques for the treatment of breast cancer in which the adrenal glands are removed along with the ovaries, thus removing *all* sources of sex steroid hormone (the adrenal glands produce a variety of steroid hormones, including all the sex hormones), the women lose virtually all interest in sex (Drellich and Waxenberg, 1966). This observation is taken to suggest that the androgens present in the adrenal glands contribute to the maintenance of sexual urges in women. And thus it seems that the sex drive in women as well as men is stimulated by androgens.

Several hypotheses have been offered which attempt to explain the observations that testosterone and other androgenic substances act as sexually stimulating agents in both males and females. For example, it has been postulated that androgens act directly on the brain. There is some experimental evidence in support of this hypothesis, for it is possible to elicit sexual activity in laboratory animals by implanting the sex steroids in the brain. Another way for the androgens to stimulate the sex drive in both sexes would be for the hormone to sensitize the genital organs in some way which would ultimately stimulate the person to seek sexual outlets. In a man this kind of hormone-induced genital sensitization could manifest itself by the build-up of seminal fluid in the seminal vesicles and the prostate gland. With the accumulation of seminal fluid, a man would be stimulated to seek ejaculatory release. In the female androgens may sensitize the clitoris, which is known to be an androgen-sensitive structure, and in this way somehow elevate sexual desires in women. It has also been proposed that androgens may increase the flow of blood into the pelvic vasculature, which could give rise to feelings of sexual tension emanating from the pelvic region.

SEXUAL
RELATIONS

The release of biologically generated sexual tensions and the sexual expression of feeling can be achieved by engaging in sexual relations with members of the opposite sex (heterosexual relations), by engaging in sexual relations with members of the same sex (homosexual relations), and by self-stimulation of the genital organs and other sexually sensitive organs of the body (masturbation). Theoretically, each of these forms of sexual outlet is capable of providing sexual gratification. However, the most common form of human sexual expression is, by far, heterosexual coitus (Ford and Beach, 1953). Although many people engage in various forms of noncoital sexual activity, the majority prefer heterosexual intercourse as their primary mode of sexual release (Table 3-1).

HETEROSEXUAL
RELATIONS

One of the major reasons that heterosexual intercourse is the most common form of sexual activity is that societies tend to encourage their members to engage in heterosexual coitus while exercising rigid control over other forms of sexual activity, if not prohibiting them altogether. Moreover, most societies attempt to channel sexual relations to take place within the societally defined context of marriage. Thus, heterosexual relations between the yet unmarried (premarital intercourse) and sexual relations between married people and partners other than their spouses (extramarital intercourse) are often prohibited in many societies, as are homosexual relations and masturbation. Virtually all societies regulate sexual activity believed to be a threat to the prestige of marriage as a social institu-

TABLE 3.1
PERCENTAGE OF TOTAL SEXUAL OUTLET BY SOURCE

Male (age 21-40)		Female (age 21-40)	
Masturbation	approx. 15%	Masturbation	approx. 17%
Nocturnal orgasm	5	Nocturnal orgasm	2
Petting	2	Petting	2
Coitus, any	75-80	Coitus, any	70
premarital	10	premarital	6
marital	75	marital	60
extramarital	5	extramarital	5
postmarital	2	postmarital	6
Homosexual	8	Homosexual	4
Total autosexual	20	Total autosexual	17
Total heterosexual	70	Total heterosexual	80
Total homosexual	10	Total homosexual	4

SOURCE   A. C. Kinsey et al., *Sexual Behavior in the Human Male* (Philadelphia: Saunders, 1948), p. 488 and A. C. Kinsey et al., *Sexual Behavior in the Human Female* (Philadelphia: Saunders, 1953), p. 561.

tion or the stability of the marital unit. The rules governing sexual expression may vary in detail from society to society, and their authority may be derived from either religious fiat, cultural norm, or legal sanction.

MARITAL AND EXTRAMARITAL SEXUAL RELATIONSHIPS
Of the many reasons that people marry—economic security, social status, the desire to have children, availability of a sex partner, and the desire to love and be loved—the most common for Americans is the latter, the desire to give and receive love and to fulfill one's emotional needs within a love relationship. When American husbands and wives are asked why they married, their most frequent response is that they were in love. It should be noted that love is not the traditional reason for marriage. In former times people married primarily to have children and to cooperate in economic support. The interpersonal relationship between the partners was rarely of fundamental concern. Often the marriage partners did not even choose each other; the marriages were arranged by their respective

families. This is no longer the case in the majority of present-day marriages. Because the marital relationship has shifted from a predominantly childbearing-socioeconomic relationship to one in which the emotional gratification of the individuals involved is of primary importance, people demand the option of choosing the partner who they feel holds the most promise of providing a close relationship which is mutually satisfying and emotionally supportive.

The expectation that marriage is to be primarily an intimate relationship and only secondarily a familial one tends to place great emphasis on the sexual relations between the marital partners. In a marriage where personal involvement is little expected or even desired, the fundamental role of sex is to create children, relieve sexual tensions, and provide physical pleasure. In a marriage where emotional closeness is the goal, sex not only provides a context for the giving and receiving of sensual gratification but is also an important avenue of communication within the marriage. The sexual relationship becomes a physical manifestation of the personal, emotional relationship between the marital partners.

Because sex is a highly effective form of interpersonal communication it often acts as a "weathervane" of marital harmony and happiness. If people have a healthy, happy marriage this situation can be reflected in a satisfying and fulfilling sexual relationship. If a marriage is strained, however, the partners may be unhappy, and their sexual relationship dissatisfying or even nonexistent. Some couples have mistakenly tried to employ the frequency that they have sexual intercourse as a measure of sexual and marital adjustment and satisfaction. They worry whether their frequency of sexual relations is "normal." What these people fail to realize is that normal frequency of intercourse is established by each couple based upon their mutual needs for sexual release. Some couples find daily intercourse the most satisfying while others are happy to have sex only once or twice a month. The frequency of sexual intercourse is not the important factor, rather, it is the quality of the sexual experience that should be of concern. Sex should be physically satisfying to be sure, but it should also bring personal closeness and strengthen the emotional relationship.

One of the traditional ideals of the American marriage is that married people have sexual relations exclusively with their mates. Marital partners are expected to be "faithful" to one another, meaning that they will not have sexual intercourse with other people. In some marriage ceremonies the partners explicitly vow "to cleave only to one another" or to "forsake all others." Even if such promises are not made verbally, they are nevertheless implicitly understood as part of the marriage contract because extramarital sex is strongly prohibited in our culture. Sexual intercourse with a person other than one's spouse is a violation of the Seventh Commandment, and in many states it is considered a crime.

Marriage promises, custom, and religious and secular law notwithstanding, about one half of the married men in the United States and about one fourth of the married women admit to having sexual relations outside their marriage (Kinsey et al., 1948, 1953). Oftentimes the extramarital relationships are brief liaisons formed strictly to experience physical sexual gratification with a new partner. Such relationships are usually entered into for the purpose of having a new and perhaps exciting sexual experience. It is a way some married people attempt to add variety to their sexual lives after having restricted themselves to sexual intercourse with the same partner for many years.

Some people have sexual relations outside their marriage because the emotional relationship with their mate has either changed by not meeting premarital expectations, or has deteriorated to the point that the partners have difficulty communicating with one another on any level. In these instances emotional need fulfillment is no longer obtained from the spouse and so a person looks to other individuals to fill the emotional "void." It is interesting to note that some spouses are willing to tolerate the brief sexual liaisons of their mates if they are for sexual reasons only. But most are unwilling to accept competitive emotional attachments which present a threat to the marriage.

In only a few societies are there no restrictions whatsoever on the sexual behavior of married people except for the taboo against incest. In some societies a particular type of extramarital sex is allowed, but the situations in which it can take place are carefully described. For example, an Eskimo man may "lend" his wife for the purpose of sexual intercourse to a visiting man who is without his own wife. In the Siriono society of South America, sexual relations are permitted with mates of siblings and siblings of mates.

HOMOSEXUAL
RELATIONSHIPS

Sexual relations between members of the same sex are referred to as homosexual. Both males and females can take part in homosexual relations, but in American society men tend to have homosexual experiences more often than women; approximately one third of the men are believed to have had some homosexual contact sometime in their lives, while the incidence for women is about half that for men (Kinsey et al., 1948, 1953). Not all of those who admit to having had homosexual experiences are exclusively homosexual; the majority of them have only a transitory experience with a same-sexed partner, oftentimes simply because a partner of the opposite sex is unavailable. Such may be the circumstance of prisoners, students in single-sex schools, people in the armed forces, men on ships, and adolescents who are forbidden heterosexual outlets. When heterosexual relations do become available to these people, their homosexual contacts usually cease. Only about 4 percent of males and 2 percent of females are reported to restrict sexual relations exclusively to members of their own sex (Kinsey at al., 1953). These people are given the name "homosexuals." They are people who are "motivated in adult life by a definite preferential erotic attraction to members of the same sex and who usually (but not necessarily) engage in overt sexual relations with them" (Marmor, 1964). Moreover, many homosexuals are actually unable to form deep emotional attachments to members of the opposite sex.

Homosexual practices involve many of the techniques of sexual stimulation indicative of heterosexual stimulation, except, of course, actual sexual intercourse. Homosexual relations in males usually consist of manual-genital and oral-genital stimulation and anal intercourse. Female homosexual relations involve mutual stimulation of the breasts and genital region by both mouth and hand.

The interpersonal sexual relationships of male and female homosexuals appear to differ. Male homosexuals tend to become involved in casual and frequent homosexual encounters, whereas female homosexuals tend to establish rather stable partnerships (Saghir et al., 1969). Even in male homosexual relationships in which an emotional attachment exists between the partners, exclusivity with respect to sexual partners is rarely practiced. In the majority of these relationships the partners participate in several homosexual encounters. This is in contrast to most female homosexual relationships in which sexual exclusivity is usually practiced.

MASTURBATION

Masturbation is self-stimulation to effect sexual arousal usually to the point of orgasm. Although considered a sexual perversion in nearly all Western societies, masturbation is nevertheless a common sexual activity in most human cultures. It has even been observed to occur in nonhuman animals such as the chimpanzee and the elephant. Kinsey's study of American sexual behavior reported that nearly all males (92 percent) have masturbatory experiences by age 20 and that about two thirds of the females employ masturbation as a sexual outlet, with the greatest incidence occurring after age 25 (Kinsey et al., 1953).

The most common masturbatory techniques used by both men and women involve manual manipulation of the genital region. For males this includes rubbing or stroking the penis, while for females it involves manual stimulation of the entire mons area, particularly the clitoral region, the vaginal labia, with occasional vaginal insertions. Few women directly stimulate the clitoris due to that organ's extreme sensitivity when a woman is sexually excited (Masters and Johnson, 1966). Autostimulation of the sexually sensitive nongenital areas such as the breasts and anal region are additional masturbatory techniques. There are also reports of women who are able to fantasy to orgasm (Kinsey et al., 1953; Masters and Johnson, 1970).

Some people believe masturbation is an expression of a pathological personality, but the frequency with which it occurs suggests that it is a normal human sexual outlet, employed as a means of sexual tension release when interpersonal sexual contact is not possible. This is believed to be the reason for the high incidence of masturbation among adolescent males, as they are forbidden in our society to engage in heterosexual intercourse until they are older (Marmor, 1969). Masturbation is also frequently employed by single adults who have no formal or regular sexual outlet and also by married adults who have irregular or nonexistent sexual relations within their marriage.

Masturbation is often accompanied by sexual fantasies. Approximately 75 percent of the males who masturbate and nearly 50 percent of the women who masturbate report that sexual fantasy occurs with masturbation. It is believed that such fantasizing creates for the individual the imaginary experiences of an actual interpersonal sexual relationship. The exact nature of the fantasized relationship or experience is believed to reflect aspects of the individual's personality (Bonime, 1969).

A number of personal harmful physical effects are rumored to occur because of masturbation. Among these are loss of hair, insanity, pimples, warts, unhappiness in marriage, and sterility. There is absolutely no medical evidence for such beliefs. There does seem to be differing opinion as to the possible harmful psychological effects of masturbation. One school of thought holds that masturbation, by providing a unitary or solitary sexual experience, is prohibiting the consummation of more "natural" heterosexual interpersonal experiences. On the other hand, masturbation can serve as a beneficial release of built-up sexual tensions. This is sometimes called the pacifier effect (Marmor, 1969). It can be seen to occur among individuals at times of higher than normal tension when masturbation is used as a means of tension release through sexual orgasm.

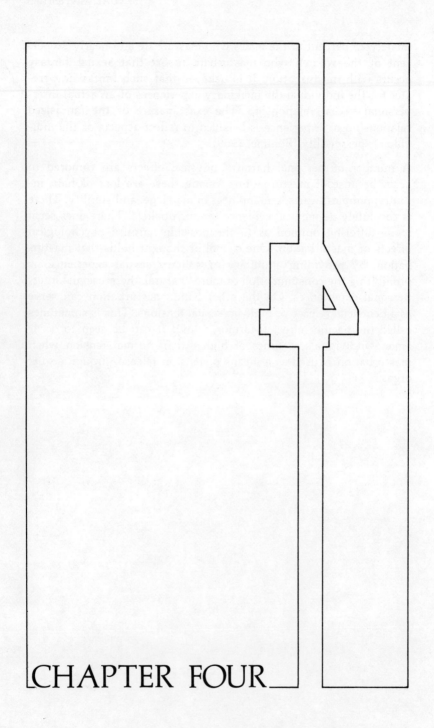

CHAPTER FOUR

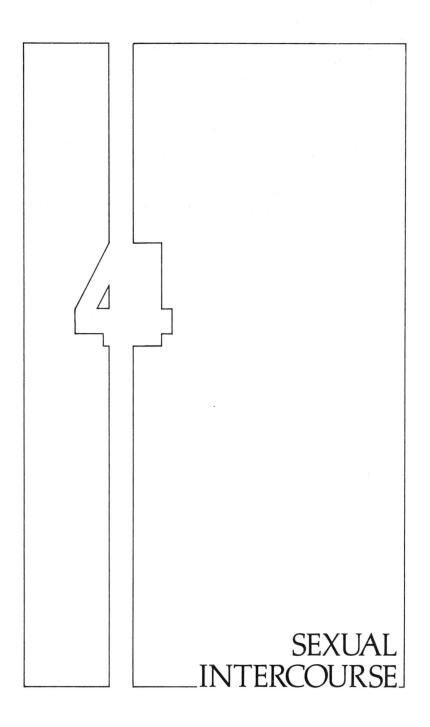

4

SEXUAL
INTERCOURSE

The sex act involves the mutual exchange of sexual stimulation to produce sexual pleasure and excitement. There are certain areas of the human body which, when properly stimulated, produce erotic arousal. These sexually sensitive areas are referred to as *erogenous zones*. The most sensitive erogenous zones are the genital organs—the clitoris of the woman and the penis of the man. Other erogenous areas include the vaginal lips, breasts, lips of the mouth, parts of the ears, and the anal region. When the erogenous zones are stimulated by either gentle caressing, kissing, or gentle forms of pressure contact, a number of physiological changes take place. These bodily responses to sexual stimulation involve the tightening of the muscles, especially in the pelvic areas, and the swelling of the genital organs and other erogenous parts of the body such as the breasts. As sexual stimulation is continued, the overall physiological response in both sexes manifests itself in faster breathing rates, a higher heart rate, and a rise in blood pressure (Figure 4-1). In conjunction with the changes in body physiology, sexual stimulation also produces feelings of intense pleasure and excitement.

When the sexual tensions increase to a certain point they are at once released in a massive pleasurable outburst involving the person's entire body; this is orgasm. *Orgasm* is a multifaceted psychophysiological phenomenon which occurs at the peak of sexual stimulation in both men and women. Physiologically, orgasm is the release of the muscular and vascular tensions which build up during the preorgasmic phases of a sexual episode. It is the release of these tensions which make the orgasm so pleasurable. Orgasm in the male is accompanied by ejaculation, and so it is important that a male be stimulated to orgasm if fertilization is to occur. Women do not ejaculate or ovulate at orgasm, so the reproductive significance of female orgasm is less obvious (see below).

It is useful to consider the human sex act as occurring in four phases: (1) the precopulatory phase, when the first stages of physical contact between sexual partners produce the first sexual responses; (2) the copulatory phase, when intromission takes place and further sexual stimulation is brought about by active copulation; (3) the orgasmic phase; (4) the postorgasmic phase, when elevated levels of sexual tension subside and the body physiologially returns to normal.

PRECOPULATORY PHASE

In the precopulatory phase of the sex act, the partners stimulate each other's erogenous zones in a variety of ways in order to increase the levels of sexual excitement and tension and to bring each other toward the climactic experience of orgasm. In America and Northern Europe kissing is perhaps the most common method of initiating a sexual episode. Kissing in this totally sexual context may sometimes take the form of so-called French kissing or deep kissing where the tongue is inserted into the mouth of the kissing partner and the inner surfaces of the lips and mouth are stimulated. Even in societies where rubbing noses is the predominant form of affectionate expression, French kissing may be part of the sex act. During the more intense moments of a sexual encounter, oral stimulation can diversify to biting the partner's lips and mouth and nibbling or sucking on the ear lobes and neck.

Another precopulatory activity which occurs in a significant number of human cultural groups is the gentle fondling, kissing, or sucking of the female breasts. This type of sexual stimulation is virtually unique among humans because the breasts of nonhuman mammals are prominent only when the females suckle newborn young. The breasts of human females become prominent during adolescence and remain so for life, even when women are not breast-feeding. It has been suggested that human females evolved with perpetually prominent breasts because males found the sight and touch of the breasts erotically arousing and therefore chose well-breasted women as sexual partners (Morris, 1966). It is also possible that the tactile sensitivity of the breasts created the desire among females for sexual activity and they mated more often. The breasts respond to tactile stimulation by enlarging, often becoming approximately 25 percent greater in size (Figure 4–2). They also become firmer. The nipples may become erect, particularly if oral stimulation is applied, and the color of the area around the nipples may darken.

A more direct precopulatory activity is the stimulation of the

65

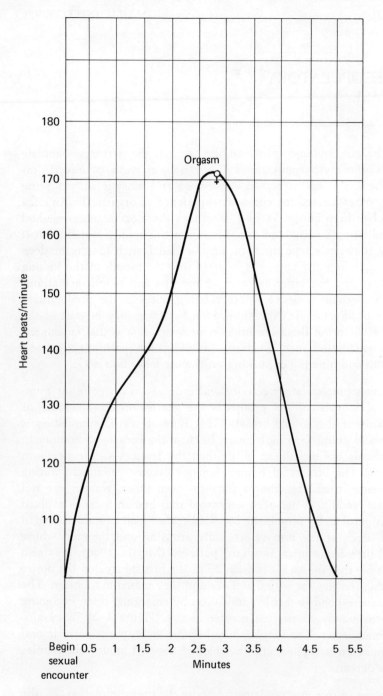

FIGURE 4-1
Changes in heart rate in a male and a female during sexual intercourse.

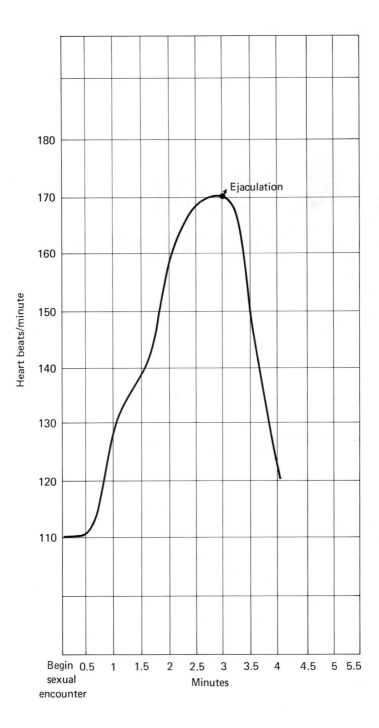

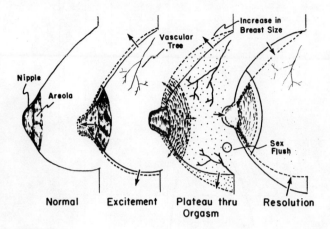

Normal   Excitement   Plateau thru   Resolution
                        Orgasm

FIGURE 4-2

Enlargement of the breast due to sexual excitation. From W. Masters and V. Johnson, *Human Sexual Response* (Boston: Little, Brown, 1966). Reprinted by permission.

external genitalia. This type of sexual activity is common to some animal species as well as humans. A male dog, for example, will lick the vulva of a female in heat, and female monkeys sometimes manipulate the penis of a prospective mate before copulation. In the human sex act both partners often participate in genital stimulation. The female partner may rub or stroke her partner's penis, and the male partner may explore with his hand the entire genital area of his mate, including the vagina, the vaginal lips, and especially the clitoris. It is not uncommon, and certainly not unnatural, for sex partners to kiss, suck, or even gently bite the genitals of their mates in order to increase the level of sexual excitement. Such activity may bring some people directly to orgasm without actual copulation taking place. Oral stimulation of the female genitals is called cunnilingus, and its counterpart, the oral stimulation of the penis, is called fellatio. Occasionally sex partners will participate in simultaneous oral-genital stimulation referred to as "soixante-neuf" or sixty-nine. This practice may serve to heighten sexual excitement in two ways, for not only do the partners receive physical stimulation but also the gratification of effecting intense sexual pleasure in the sex partner.

The result of sexual stimulation in the precopulatory phase of the sex act is that both sexes become physiologicaly prepared for active

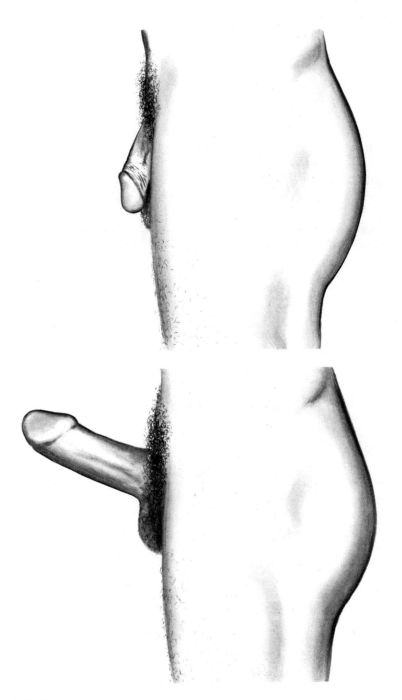

FIGURE 4-3
Erection of the penis.

sexual intercourse. The primary physiological response of the male to effective sexual stimulation is erection of the penis. Since the human male's penis is normally flaccid, penile erection is mandatory if sexual intercourse is to occur. The penis could not accomplish the pistonlike thrusting necessary to stimulate the male and female to orgasm if it remained flaccid. Thus, when a male becomes sexually aroused, regardless of the form of sexual stimulation, the penile arteries dilate and the amount of blood flowing into the penis exceeds the amount of blood flowing out, thus causing the penis to fill with blood and become hard and erect (Figure 4-3). This pronounced change in the male anatomy occurs very rapidly, usually within a few seconds after a man is exposed to any sexually arousing stimulus.

For a woman the major response to effective sexual stimulation is the appearance of lubricating secretions within the vagina. These secretions also appear rapidly after the first sexually arousing stimulus, normally within 10 to 30 seconds. There have been many suggestions as to the source of vaginal secretions, including the cervix and the Bartholin's glands, but the actual source appears to be the vaginal walls themselves (Masters and Johnson, 1966). Photographic studies of the vaginal lubrication response show that the vaginal secretions first appear as drops of mucuslike material which exude from the walls of the vagina, a phenomenon similar to the appearance of beads of sweat on the forehead (Figure 4–4). Increased sexual stimulation causes the "sweating phenomenon" to continue and the many drops eventually coalesce to form a smooth lubricating surface inside the entire vagina. The vaginal secretions do not appear to come from any special glands within the vaginal walls, but are probably produced as a result of the prominent congestion of the blood vessels in the pelvic areas which results from sexual arousal. Vaginal secretions are important in sexual intercourse because they lubricate the vagina to allow the friction from penile thrusting to proceed smoothly and without pain.

Because the source of vaginal lubricant is the vagina itself, women who have had their ovaries or uterus removed for health reasons are still capable of vaginal lubrication and therefore normal sexual activity. Menopause will not impede the ability of women to produce vaginal secretions, although the rapidity with which they

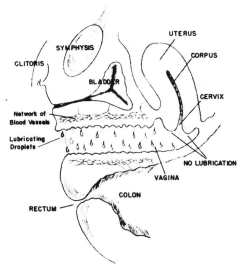

FIGURE 4-4
Lubrication reaction of the vagina due to sexual excitation. From W. Masters and V. Johnson, *Human Sexual Response* (Boston: Little, Brown, 1966). Reprinted by permission.

appear may wane with advancing age due to the decline in sex hormone production.

In addition to producing lubricating secretions, the vagina responds to sexual stimulation by enlarging, and in so doing it becomes prepared to accept the penis. In the normal, unstimulated state the vaginal walls may touch, but when a woman becomes sexually excited the walls of the inner two thirds of the vagina separate to create a vaginal barrel enlarged by approximately 2 cm in length and 4 cm in width (Figure 4–5).

The vaginal lips, like the vaginal barrel, also respond to sexual stimulation as if they were preparing to accept the penis. Sexual stimulation causes the labia majora to flatten back, away from the body midline, which exposes the vagina for penile insertion. At the same time the labia minora become engorged with blood and increase two to three times in diameter. This causes the normally

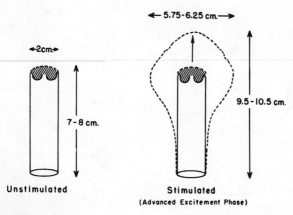

FIGURE 4-5
Enlargement of the vagina due to sexual excitation. From W. Masters and V. Johnson, *Human Sexual Response* (Boston: Little, Brown, 1966). Reprinted by permission.

inner-lying labia minora to protrude past the outer, now folded back labia majora.

Along with the swelling, the minor labia undergo a noticeable color change, ranging from bright pink to a red or wine color. This color change is called the "sex skin," and it is considered a certain sign that a woman is sexually excited (Masters and Johnson, 1966). The sex skin also appears in some nonhuman primate species during mating periods and serves as a signal for the male that the female is ready to copulate. The sex skin response of human females could be a vestige of their primate ancestry.

The clitoris also responds rapidly to sexual stimulation in much the same way as its homologous organ in the male, the penis. Like the penis, the clitoral response to sexual stimulation is to engorge with blood, which causes the glans portion of the clitoris to swell and the clitoral shaft to elongate and increase in diameter. The clitoral response occurs shortly after the vaginal lubrication response, but the extent and rapidity of the response depends upon the type of stimulation employed. The clitoris responds most rapidly and extensively to direct manipulation, either by hand or mouth, and more slowly and less overtly to coitus, breast manipulation, and fantasy (Masters and Johnson, 1966).

COPULATORY PHASE

The copulatory phase of the sex act begins when the male inserts his penis in the female's vagina. Although most nonhuman animals copulate by the male entering the female from the rear, the most frequently employed human coital position is one in which the sex partners face each other. The most common face-to-face position is the "female supine position" (Figure 4–6). In this coital position, the female lies on her back with her thighs separated and the male mounts her from atop, sometimes supporting his weight on his knees and elbows. Most American couples use the female supine position in the majority of their coital experiences (Kinsey et al., 1953).

Other commonly used variations of the face-to-face coital posture include the lateral coital position (Figure 4–7), or the female superior position, where the female sits astride the male (Figure 4–8). Of the commonly used coital positions, only the lateral and female superior positions allow for any primary stimulation of the clitoral area (Masters and Johnson, 1970), for they bring the pubic symphyses of the partners in close opposition. Many times couples prefer these positions for they give the female more control over the rate and degree of coital stimulation through the controlled movement of her hips. The lateral position is especially effective in this regard, giving the female control over the rate and intensity of her sexual response and giving the male more control over the timing of ejaculation.

There are numerous coital positions which people use as variations to the more frequently used postures. Some of these positions do not require that the partners lie down but rather that one or both sit or stand. Another variation is to have vaginal entry from the rear. In this position the penis does not stroke the clitoral area but there is significant secondary stimulation due to tractions on the labial structures as a result of penile thrusting. Also, vaginal penetration from the rear can be very deep, even to the point of contact with the cervix, which some people find very stimulating.

The sensations derived from sexual intercourse are virtually all

73

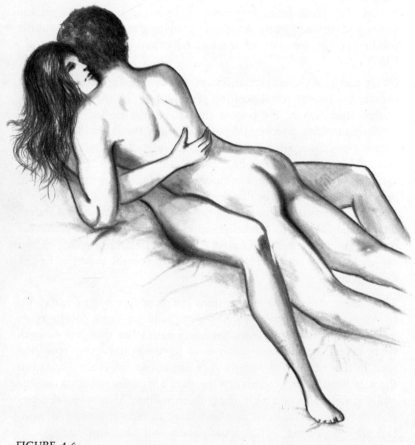

FIGURE 4-6
Female supine coital position.

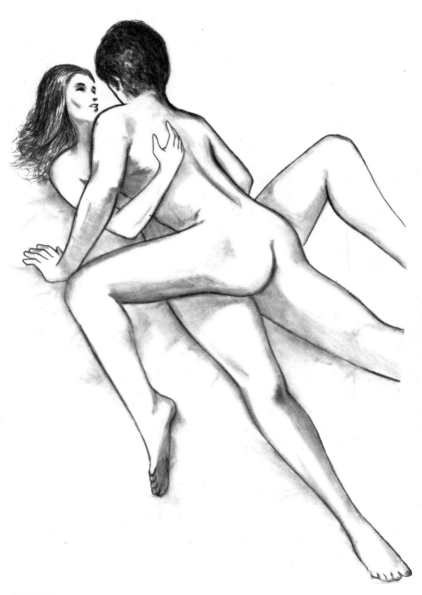

FIGURE 4-7
Lateral coital position.

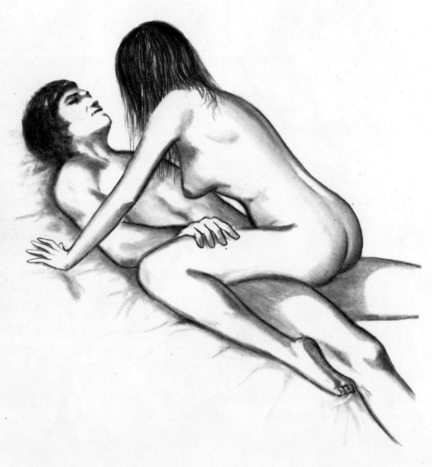

FIGURE 4-8
Female superior coital position.

pelvic in origin, emanating mostly from the penis or the clitoris. The main source of penile stimulation during intercourse results from the friction on the penis caused by the rhythmic and piston-like thrusting of the penis in and out of the vagina. The female's sensations come from stimulation of the clitoral area even though the clitoris is withdrawn into its protective foreskin by the time actual coitus begins (Masters and Johnson, 1966). Since direct touching of the clitoris is not possible, and may even be irritating to some women if attempted, stimulation during sexual intercourse arises from penile thrusting exerting a push-and-pull on the labial structures and over the clitoral area.

In addition to direct genital stimulation during coitus, many people will further excite their partners with deep erotic kisses, manipulation of other erogenous areas, and the exchange of vocal signs of pleasure, love, and tenderness.

ORGASMIC PHASE

Orgasm in the male is preceded by the sensation that ejaculation is going to occur and that it cannot be stopped. The sensation of the inevitability of ejaculation occurs within two to four seconds before the actual onset of the orgasm. During the ejaculatory episode the male's psychic focus is on the expulsion of seminal fluid as he experiences strong contractions of the pelvic musculature.

At the onset of the female orgasm, women tend to feel a sensation of stoppage with an accompanying intense clitoral-pelvic awareness (Masters and Johnson, 1966). This is soon followed by a feeling of a "suffusion of warmth" and then the consuming awareness of the ensuing orgasmic contractions, especially of the outer one third of the vagina.

When orgasm does occur, the muscular tensions which accumulated during the entire sexual episode are released through involuntary contractions primarily in the pelvic area. In the male, contractions of the pelvic muscles help expel the seminal fluid from its source in the genital ducts out the penile urethra. In the female, orgasm brings about contractions of the uterus and vagina. In both sexes additional orgasmic contractions also take place in the rectal sphincter and the gluteus muscles of the buttocks, and sometimes a facial grimace appears due to the release of muscular tensions in the head and neck.

In both the male and the female the initial orgasmic contractions occur at intervals of 0.8 seconds (Masters and Johnson, 1966). There are usually four of these regular contractions in the male and as many as eight in the female. After this initial orgasmic release, the contractions become less frequent and occur thereafter at irregular intervals.

POSTORGASMIC PHASE

Once a male has ejaculated, the penis usually becomes flaccid, and the man is unable to continue with sexual intercourse for a period of time, the length of which depends upon his age and the degree of his sexual excitement at the time. In adolescent males, the ability to achieve an erection after orgasm can occur rapidly, perhaps within a few minutes after ejaculation. Older males, however, usually require a longer period to recover erection ability. This time period is usually a half hour to an hour for most men, and up to days for some others. In contrast to males, some women are able to experience more than one orgasm during a single coital episode.

The duration of sexual intercourse is usually determined by the time the male takes to reach orgasm. In other animals the entire sex act can be concluded in a rather short period of time, as the male is quick to insert his penis into the vagina, ejaculate, and withdraw. Sexual intercourse among baboons, for example, may take only 15 seconds.

Quite the opposite behavior is considered normal for human beings. If a male inserts his penis and ejaculates immediately, before his partner has been stimulated to a high degree and is ready for orgasm, the male is considered to be sexually inadequate. Unfortunately such a phenomenon is all too common, for many men seem to have never learned, or they do not appreciate the fact, that women are capable of enjoying sex at least as much as and perhaps more than men. In many instances it is often totally unsatisfying for a woman to engage in sexual contact and begin the crescendo of sexual excitement, only to have her partner ejaculate and break off contact before she has reached orgasm. With a reasonable period of precoital stimulation, many women find a three- to five-minute coital interlude sufficient to effect at least one orgasm.

Some people feel that orgasmic release should occur simultaneously in both partners if the utmost pleasure is to be derived from coitus. While this may be true for some couples, it is nevertheless important to realize that a sexual relationship may still be satisfying and entirely healthy if the partners arrive at orgasm at different times in the sex act. It should also be noted that a satisfying sexual relationship does not require that both partners reach orgasm in every coital episode.

From a biological point of view, the characteristics of human sexuality exist because they in some way mediate reproduction, and this is presumably true of orgasm. The reproductive significance of the male orgasm is obvious, since ejaculation is necessary if fertilization is going to take place. On the other hand, there is no obvious reproductive significance of orgasm in women. It has been suggested that the female orgasm is important in reproduction because the uterine contractions which occur during orgasm help propel sperm through the uterus to the uterine tubes, either by creating suctions in the uterus or by creating peristaltic motions in the fluids on the inner surface of the uterus which would aid sperm mobility.

Another explanation of the possible function of the female orgasm takes note of the fact that of all mammalian females, only humans walk in the upright position and postulates that the ability of human females to experience orgasm has evolved as a consequence of bipedalism. The idea is that the female orgasm aids fertilization because it fatigues the woman to the degree that she will not walk away from a sexual encounter immediately after insemination, as do most other mammalian females. If a woman walks soon after her partner has ejaculated, some of the ejaculate certainly escapes the vagina. Since it is known that conception is difficult if low

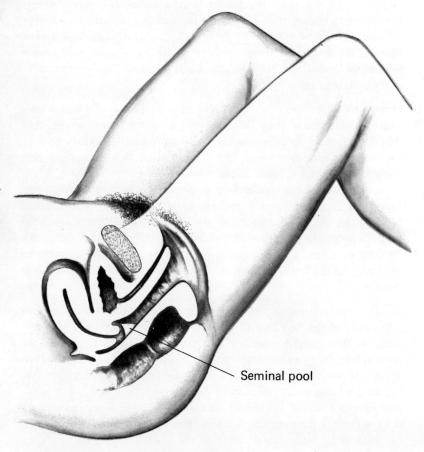

Seminal pool

FIGURE 4-9
Seminal pool in the vagina after ejaculation.

numbers of sperm are ejaculated into the vagina, it is reasonable to assume that if some of the ejaculate were lost because the woman stood up after intercourse, the number of sperm necessary to effect fertilization might be insufficient. Thus it would seem important that a woman remain in a horizontal position after the male ejaculates, preferably on her back, so that the seminal fluid will pool in the upper end of the vagina and increase the probability of sperm entering the uterus (Figure 4–9).

While it is true that the extensive muscular contractions which are part of the female orgasm may in some way increase the probability of successful fertilization, it is also true that orgasm is extremely pleasurable, and therefore its significance in human reproduction may not be any direct physical aid to fertilization, but may be that it increases the frequency with which women desire sex. By increasing the pleasure in the female sex act, women are motivated to engage in sex more often.

There has been much confusion about the female orgasm stemming from the idea that there are two distinct forms of female orgasmic response, the clitoral orgasm and the vaginal orgasm. The existence of the two separate orgasms is based upon the belief that the clitoris is a vestigial penis devoid of any major feminine qualities. Thus, women who focus on the clitoris in their sexual response are considered to be sexually "immature." This theory goes on to state that only when a woman has matured to the full limits of her sexuality will she cease to experience clitoral orgasms and enjoy vaginal orgasms exclusively. A careful study, however, has shown that there is no physiological difference in female orgasm regardless of the psychic sensations which accompany it (Masters and Johnson, 1966). There seems to be no basis for believing that there are two distinct types of female orgasm.

SEXUAL INADEQUACY

A person's physical ability to participate in sexual intercourse involves the coordination of a number of physiological, psychological, and interpersonal factors. Included in these factors are the general level of health and vitality, the functional state of the sexual anatomy, one's values and attitudes about sex, one's feelings about one's self and about others, and the nature of the relationship with the sex partner. Those who enjoy a vigorous, active, and satisfying sex life tend to be physically healthy and tend to hold positive attitudes about the ways they express themselves sexually. Some people, however, because of poor health, malfunctioning sexual organs, or negative attitudes about sex or their sex partner, are physically unable to take part in sexual intercourse in a normal satisfying way. The various difficulties that people have which impede the attainment of normal sexual functioning are called sexual inadequacies.

One of the major sexual inadequacies to occur in men is the inability to achieve an erection or the inability to maintain an erection long enough to have sexual intercourse. This form of sexual inadequacy is called *impotence.* Impotence can be classified as either primary or secondary. Primary impotence refers to a condition in which a man has never in his life been able to attain an erection for the purpose of taking part in sexual intercourse. Secondary impotence refers to a condition in which a man loses his ability to get an erection after having experienced a time in which he was potent and capable of sexual relations. Of the two forms of impotence, secondary impotence is more prevalent.

It is not uncommon for a man who is unable to achieve and maintain an erection when attempting to engage in sexual intercourse to be able to get an erection during sleep, by dreaming about something sexually arousing, or by having sexual fantasies. He may even be able to produce an erection and masturbate to ejaculation. Some men are impotent only with certain women. For example, there are men who are impotent with their own wives but who are fully capable of having sexual intercourse with other women.

Another form of male sexual inadequacy is called *premature ejaculation.* In this instance the man does not have problems achieving an erection, but instead has difficulty withholding ejaculation for a reasonable period of time after coitus has begun. In premature ejaculation the man ejaculates either before the insertion of the penis into the vagina or shortly after vaginal insertion. This results in a coital episode that is all too brief for most couples. The woman has been denied the opportunity to be coitally stimulated to orgasm, and both she and her partner lose the opportunity to experience a form of communication that is unique among human transactions.

In women, sexual inadequacies include experiencing pain during sexual intercourse, the inability to achieve orgasm, and the inability to accept the penis into the vagina. This latter form of female sexual inadequacy is called *vaginismus*, and it occurs when the muscles that surround the outer one third of the vagina involuntarily constrict and make penetration by the penis impossible, or very painful if attempted. The constriction of the vaginal opening in vaginismus is often not limited to situations involving sexual intercourse. Some women with vaginismus are unable to use a tampon during menstruation or undergo a routine medical examination of the vagina and cervix.

The causes of sexual inadequacies in both men and women can be many and varied. Some of the causes are physiological and some are psychological. Many diseases, for example, can impair one's ability to perform the sex act (Table 4–1). This is particularly true of diseases of the endocrine (hormone) system and nervous system, both of which are intimately involved in the control of proper sexual functioning. Other organic causes of sexual inadequacy are infection and inflammation of the genitalia or injury to the sex organs. Some factors which affect one's psychological abilities to participate in sexual intercourse are anxiety, fatigue, depression, and excessive use of alcohol, barbiturates, morphine, and heroin. Aging can also contribute to the loss of sexual ability, although many older people continue to enjoy sex in their sixties and seventies.

One of the most common causes of sexual inadequacy is fear that becomes expressed as the physical inability to perform the sex act. For example, the fear of pregnancy or of contracting venereal disease can be the underlying cause of impotence in a man or vaginismus in a woman. Some people fear that they will not meet their sex partner's expectations of them as lovers and hence be judged as sexually inferior. Other fears that can become expressed as sexual inadequacies are the fear of being hurt by the penis, or of becoming "trapped" in the vagina. And some people fear losing some "part" of themselves or perhaps of losing control while engaged in sexual intercourse.

TABLE 4.1

CLASSIFICATION OF PHYSICAL CAUSES OF SECONDARY IMPOTENCE

Anatomic
Congenital deformities
Testicular fibrosis
Hydrocele

Cardiorespiratory
Angina pectoris
Myocardial infarction
Emphysema
Rheumatic fever
Coronary insufficiency
Pulmonary insufficiency

Drug Ingestion
Addictive drugs
Alcohol
Alpha-methyl-dopa
Amphetamines
Atropine
Chlordiazepoxide
Chlorprothixene
Guanethidine
Imipramine
Methantheline bromide
Monoamine oxidase inhibitors
Phenothiazines
Reserpine
Thioridazine
Nicotine (rare)
Digitalis (rare)

Endocrine
Acromegaly
Addison's disease
Adrenal neoplasms
   (with or without Cushing's
   syndrome)
Castration
Chromophobe adenoma
Craniopharyngioma
Diabetes mellitus
Eunuchoidism (including
   Klinefelter's syndrome)
Feminizing interstitial-cell
   testicular tumors

Infantilism
Ingestion of female hormones
   (estrogen)
Myxedema
Obesity
Thyrotoxicosis

Genitourinary
Perineal prostatectomy
   (frequently)
Prostatitis
Phimosis
Priapism
Suprapubic and transurethral
   prostatectomy (occasionally)
Urethritis

Hematologic
Hodgkin's disease
Leukemia, acute and chronic
Pernicious anemia

Infectious
Genital tuberculosis
Gonorrhea
Mumps

Neurologic
Amyotrophic lateral sclerosis
Cord tumors or transection
Electric shock therapy
Multiple sclerosis
Nutritional deficiencies
Parkinsonism
Peripheral neuropathies
Spina bifida
Sympathectomy
Tabes dorsalis
Temporal lobe lesions

Vascular
Aneurysm
Arteritis
Sclerosis
Thrombotic obstruction of
   aortic bifurcation

SOURCE W. Masters and V. Johnson, *Human Sexual Inadequacy* (Boston: Little, Brown, 1970), p. 184.

VENEREAL
DISEASE

Venereal diseases, commonly referred to as V.D., are bacterial infections that are nearly always contracted by means of intimate sexual contact. (The adjective "venereal" is derived from the name of the Roman goddess of love, Venus.) Hence, the most common sites of infection are the penis and urethra of the male and the vaginal labia, urethra, cervix, and vagina of the female. V.D. can, and does, occur at other sites of the body that are exposed to the infecting organisms during sexual relations such as the anus, and less commonly the mouth, fingers, and breasts.

Although there are several distinct venereal diseases, each caused by a different infecting organism, two forms of V.D. occur much more frequently than the others. These two forms are syphilis and gonorrhea, and at the present time, both are occurring at alarmingly high frequencies in the United States (Figure 4–10). This is particularly true of gonorrhea, for which nearly 700,000 new cases were reported in 1971. The cases of syphilis reported in 1971 numbered around 20,000. These statistics are all the more alarming when we realize that the cases of venereal disease reported to Public Health Departments represent only a fraction of the total number of people actually infected. Many people who contract V.D. are treated by private physicians who may not report every case they treat (even though they are required to do so by law), and many people who become infected go undetected and untreated and continue to infect their sex partners. This may be particularly true of a woman who has contracted V.D. in the vagina or on the cervix where, because of its location, the disease often goes unnoticed. The actual number of newly infected persons is therefore not known with certainty, but it is estimated that the combined total of cases of gonorrhea and syphilis is near 2 million (American Social Health Association Report, 1972).

SYPHILIS

Syphilis, also known by a variety of other names such as "siff," "lues," "pox," "old Joe," and "bad blood," is caused by the organ-

85

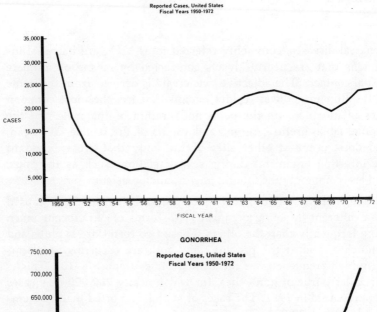

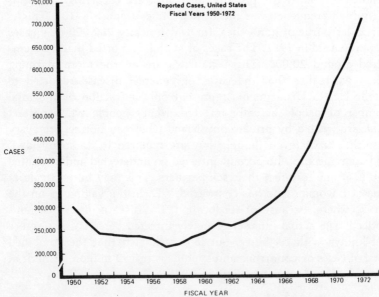

FIGURE 4-10
Incidence of syphilis and gonorrhea in the United States from 1950 to 1972.
From American Social Health Association, *Today's VD Control Problem, 1973.*
Reprinted by permission.

ism *Treponema pallidum,* a slender, spiral-shaped bacterium called a spirochete. The spread of syphilis from person to person occurs most often during sexual intercourse when organisms present on the genitalia of one partner pass to the genitalia of the other and subsequently infect him or her. The organism enters the body through breaks in the skin and then begins to multiply at the original site of entrance. Within 10 to 60 days after the initial contact, the first sign of syphilis appears usually at the site of original infection in the form of a sore or ulcer called a chancre (pronounced "shanker"). In a male a chancre most often appears on the penis and is therefore visible. In the female the chancre can appear on the labia, perineum, clitoris, or cervix. The chancre is neither itchy nor painful. It is full of treponemes, however, and therefore highly infectious. Chancres may also appear on non-genital sites of contact. Not infrequently, chancres are found in the anus as a result of anal intercourse, and they are also found on the mouth.

If the disease goes untreated the chancre heals within 3 to 8 weeks, but the person still has the infection. By this time the infecting treponemes have invaded the bloodstream and have moved throughout the entire body. In three fourths of cases, spread of the organisms leads to the outbreak of a skin rash that consists of small red spots on the trunk, arms, and legs. These lesions are also heavily laden with treponemes and therefore highly infective. The infection can also spread to the mucous membranes of the mouth. Eventually these secondary lesions heal and the disease enters a quiescent phase. The person is still infected but observable signs and symptoms are absent. This latent phase of the disease occurs about two years after the original contact.

The quiescent phase ultimately ends and a renewed period of overt symptoms appears. This is referred to as the late stage of syphilis. The manifestations of late-phase syphilis are caused by the long-term infection by treponemes, and some of the most commonly infected sites are the skin, tongue, bones, heart, and central nervous system. Approximately 10 percent of people with late-stage syphilis experience destructive effects on the heart tissue which can lead to heart failure, heart attack, and death. And nearly a third of people with late-phase syphilis have central nervous system involvement which can lead to paralysis, loss of memory, and psychosis.

In any of the stages of infection, syphilis can be diagnosed, treated, and cured. The diagnosis of syphilis is usually made by detecting the presence of *Treponema pallidum* in the blood. There are several types of blood tests for syphilis; perhaps the most well known is the Wassermann test, also known as the STS (serological test for syphilis). Other tests for syphilis include the TPI, VDRL and RPR tests. Once a diagnosis of syphilis is made a treatment regimen can be undertaken. The treatment involves administration of penicillin or an analogous antibiotic drug. Proper treatment will cure the infection, but one is likely to be susceptible to additional infections if contact with infected persons occurs again. Apparently there is little immunity built up against the disease, particularly if it is successfully treated in the early stages.

GONORRHEA

Gonorrhea, also referred to as "clap" or "a dose," is caused by the organism *Neisseria gonorrheae*, often called a gonococcus. Like syphilis, gonorrhea is spread from person to person most often through sexual contact. The disease cannot be transmitted in other ways because it cannot survive outside the body. Exposure to air kills the organisms. The route of infection occurs through the mucous membranes of the genitourinary tract that are lined by a particular type of cells (columnar epithelial cells). Thus, the most common sites of infection are the urethra, prostate, seminal vesicles, and epididymis in the male; and parts of the urethra, the cervix, and uterine tubes in the female.

Commonly, the first sign of a gonorrheal infection occurs within two to ten days after the initial exposure. Entrance of the organism into the body induces an inflammatory response in the infected person which leads to a discharge of a yellow or yellowish-green material. The discharge in males normally comes from the urethra of the penis, which gives the disease its additional slang names of "the drip" or "dew drop." Another sign in the male is painful urination. In the female, gonorrhea also produces a discharge, but it may go unnoticed. Occasionally, however, there is painful urination in females which should alert them to obtain medical attention.

If left untreated, the gonorrheal infection usually spreads into the upper genitourinary tracts in both men and women, and the resulting inflammatory response may eventually cause stricture of the male genital ducts or the female uterine tubes. In both instances the person is often left sterile.

The diagnosis of gonorrhea is usually confirmed by laboratory tests in which material from the site of the infection is examined under a microscope for the presence of gonococcal organisms. Another method of detection is to culture sample material in special culture media to determine if gonococci are present. If a person is found to have gonorrhea, he or she can be treated with penicillin or other antibiotics that will cure the infection. As with syphilis, reinfection with gonorrhea is possible if one has renewed contact with infected persons. The body builds up no resistance or immunity to the organisms. It is estimated that 15 percent of the cases of gonorrhea result from reinfections (American Social Health Association Report, 1972).

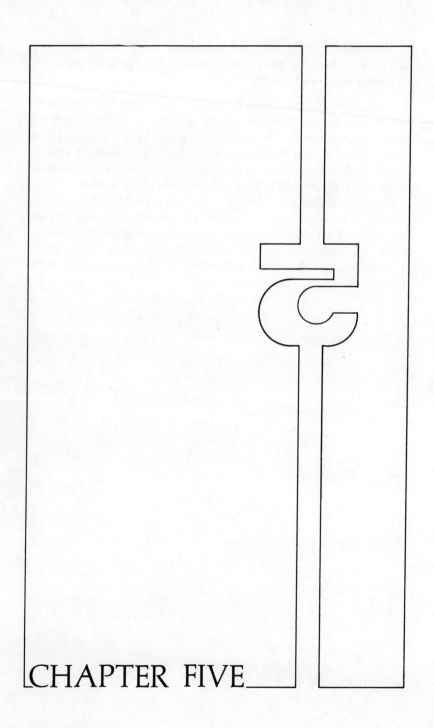

CHAPTER FIVE

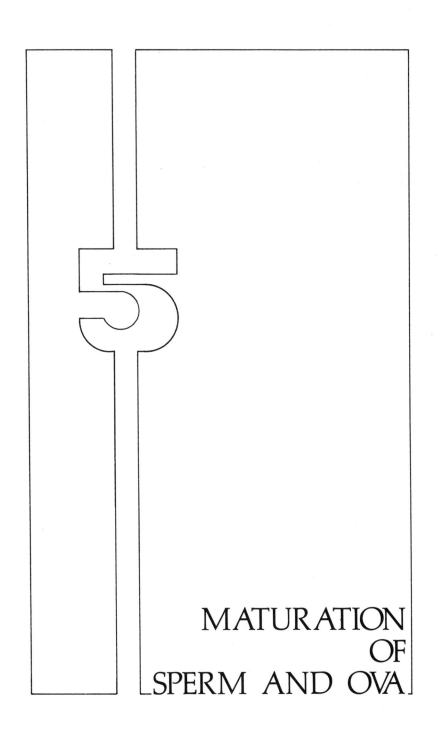

5

MATURATION
OF
SPERM AND OVA

Every human generation's genetic legacy is transmitted to the succeeding one through the fusion of specialized cells, the sperm from the male and the ovum from the female. The sperm carries 23 chromosomes which contain the father's genetic contribution to his child, and the ovum carries 23 chromosomes which are the mother's genetic contribution to her child. The genetic contributions of the parents are brought together at fertilization when the sperm and the ovum fuse, and the complete set of 46 chromosomes is formed in the zygote.

Mature human sperm (called spermatozoa) are streamlined, highly motile cells measuring about 55 or 60 microns in length. They have a sleek tadpolelike anatomy consisting of a head portion, a midpiece, and a tail (Figure 5–1). The head is a flat body shaped some-

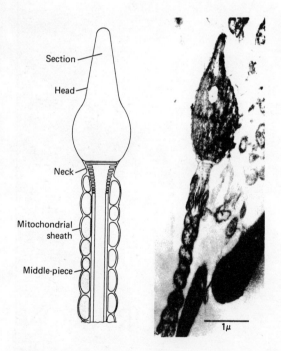

FIGURE 5-1
Electron micrograph of a human spermatozoon. From Lord Rothschild, *British Medical Journal*, 1:301 (1958).

what like an ellipse; it is about 5 microns long and 3 microns wide and contains the nucleus of the sperm cell. The midpiece is connected to the head; it is about 5 microns long and approximately 1 micron thick and contains many mitochondria, which are intracellular compartments of oxygen utilizing cells that provide the cells with energy. The tail portion is the longest of the three anatomical parts of a spermatozoon, measuring between 45 and 50 microns. It comprises the sperm cell's propulsion system. By undulating back and forth the tail gives the spermatozoon its swimming mobility.

In contrast to the elongated sperm, the mature human ovum is a larger, more robust cell (Figure 5–2). Its diameter is about 140

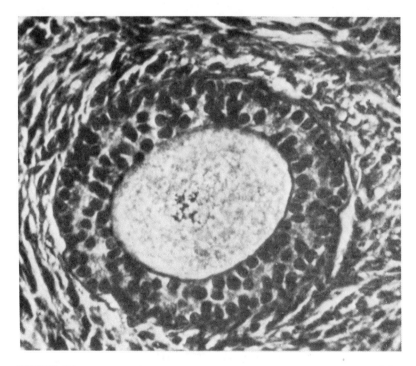

FIGURE 5-2
A human ovum. From L. Shettles, *Ovum Humanum* (New York: Haffner, 1960). Reprinted by permission.

microns. The nucleus of the ovum is near the center of the cell. Spread throughout the ovum is nutrient material, or yolk, which sustains the developing embryo in the first few days after fertilization. The ovum is enclosed in a cell membrane, and surrounding this cell membrane is a clear gelatinous membrane, approximately 5 microns thick, called the zona pellucida.

Mature sperm and ova are referred to as gametes, and the process by which they are transformed from primordial germ cells into gametes is called *gametogenesis*. Gametogenesis is characterized by two fundamental processes. One of these processes involves a change in cellular anatomy; the ovoid premature sperm cells take on the tadpolelike anatomy of mature sperm, and the premature ova grow into large cells swollen with nutrients. The second of these processes involves a reduction in the number of chromosomes in each cell from 46 to 23. The reduction in chromosome number is carried out by a process called *meiosis*.

Some simple addition will make clear the necessity for the reduction in chromosome number that takes place during meiosis. Without the halving of chromosome number in meiosis, the fusion of a sperm and an ovum containing 46 chromosomes would yield a zygote having 92 chromosomes. And when that zygote eventually developed into an adult and reproduced, it would pass its 92 chromosomes to its offspring which would then have a genetic complement of 184 chromosomes. If this were to continue, then each new generation would have twice the number of chromosomes as the one before. The halving of the number of chromosomes prevents the geometric increase in chromosome number and ensures that the number of chromosomes in each offspring is the same as the number in the parents.

Meiosis consists of several steps (Figure 5–3). The first is a replication of each chromosome to produce an exact copy. Since the number of chromosomes in human cells is 46, replication yields a cell with twice that number, or 92 chromosomes. Replication is then followed by two cellular or maturation divisions in which the chromosome number is halved each time. Thus the first maturation division yields two cells containing 46 chromosomes, and the second and final division yields four cells each with 23 chromosomes. When a mature sperm and a mature ovum fuse at fertilization, each contributes its 23 chromosomes, and so in the zygote the human species number of 46 chromosomes is restored.

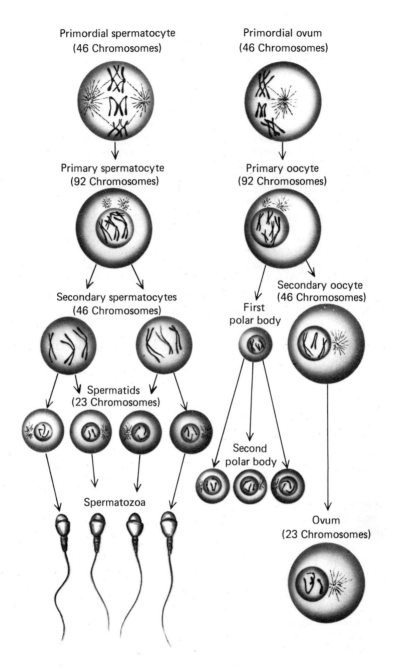

FIGURE 5-3
Meiosis in spermatozoa and ova.

HORMONAL CONTROL OF GAMETOGENESIS

The production of mature spermatozoa by males and mature ova by females is controlled by a relay of hormonal signals (Figure 5–4). The signals originate in the brain where specialized nerve cells in the hypothalamus produce and secrete certain hormones. After they are released from the brain, these hormones are shunted directly to the pituitary gland through a series of special blood vessels, and, once arriving at the pituitary gland, they induce the release of pituitary hormones into the general body circulation. For this reason the brain hormones are given the name releasing factors. There are several pituitary hormones, and the secretion of each is controlled by one or more corresponding releasing factors (Table 5–1). Two of these pituitary hormones are involved in the production of gametes in both males and females. They are *follicle*

TABLE 5.1
PITUITARY HORMONES AND CORRESPONDING RELEASING FACTORS

Pituitary hormone		Hypothalamic releasing factor	
Growth hormone, somatotrophin	GH STH	Growth hormone-releasing factor	GRF
Prolactin	none	Prolactin release-inhibiting factor	PIF
Adrenocorticotrophin	ACTH	Corticotrophin-releasing factor	CRF
Luteinizing hormone, interstitial cell stimulating hormone	LH (ICSH)	LH-releasing factor	LRF
Follicle-stimulating hormone	FSH	FSH-releasing factor	FRF
Thyroid-stimulating hormone thyrotrophin	TSH	TSH-releasing factor	TRF

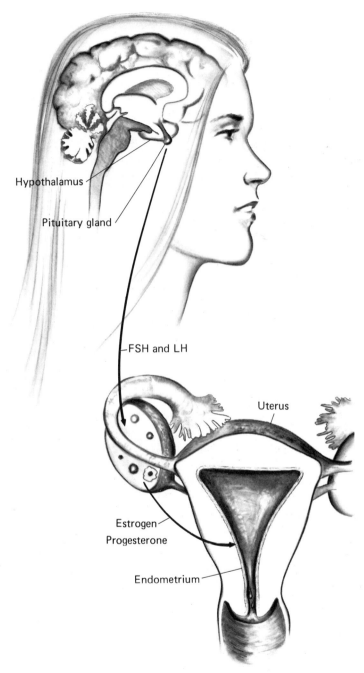

Hypothalamus

Pituitary gland

FSH and LH

Uterus

Estrogen
Progesterone

Endometrium

FIGURE 5-4
Relay of hormonal signals controlling the maturation of ova. A similar process
controls the maturation of sperm in males.

stimulating hormone (FSH) and *luteinizing hormone* (LH), and the release of these hormones from the pituitary is under the control of FSH releasing factor (FRF) and LH releasing factor (LRF).

FSH and LH are referred to as gonadotropins. Each hormone is a distinct biochemical substance with a unique chemical structure. Both FSH and LH are active in males and females. In the male, FSH is responsible for growth of the seminiferous tubules and the morphological changes that take place in sperm cells during gametogenesis. In the female, FSH is responsible for the growth of the ovarian follicle in which the ovum matures—the action from which the hormone derives its name. LH is primarily responsible for the stimulation of sex steroid production in both sexes. In the male, LH stimulates the interstitial cells of the testis to produce testosterone. (Occasionally, one can find LH referred to as interstitial cell stimulating hormone, abbreviated ICSH, because of this activity in males.) The effects of LH in the female are to stimulate the secretion of estrogen from the preovulatory follicle and estrogen and progesterone from the corpus luteum.

In many animal species the production of reproductively capable gametes in both sexes is periodic. In these species neither the males nor the females are fertile on a continual daily basis. Usually both sexes begin to produce mature gametes at one particular time of the year, with the onset of a fertile period resulting from the perception of a particular environmental stimulus. It might be a change in the amount of rainfall (salamanders), a change in the length of the day (birds), or a change in the ambient temperature (bears). If the brain interprets the environmental change as signaling the proper time for reproduction, then the cascade of hormonal signals induces the maturation and release of viable gametes. Releasing factors are secreted from the hypothalamus, which stimulate the pituitary to secrete gonadotropins which circulate through the blood to the testes or ovaries where they induce the maturation of gametes and the release of gonadal steroid hormones.

In humans, as well as many other primate species, only the female is fertile periodically. On the other hand, males are capable of producing mature spermatozoa continuously, once they have reached reproductive maturity. In these species the discharge of releasing factors from the brain does not depend on the perception of an environmental stimulus. Instead fertility is regulated internally; the males are continuously fertile and the females have recurring fertility periods controlled by internal oscillations of gonadal steroid hormone levels in the blood. In humans, the male produces about 150 million sperm per day and the female produces ova, usually one at a time, at approximately monthly intervals.

MATURATION OF SPERM

In human male embryos, primordial sperm cells can be found in the embryonic gonadal tissue about the fifth week after fertilization. These cells are referred to as *spermatogonia*. Spermatogonia do not arise directly from the embryonic gonadal tissue, but originate instead in the yolk sac of the embryo at about the fourth week of development, and then subsequently migrate to their permanent station in the tissues destined to become the testes.

During this migration and in the ensuing months after their arrival in the embryonic gonadal tissue, the spermatogonia increase in number by means of successive cellular divisions. Each cell division proceeds through a process called *mitosis* in which the original cell doubles its chromosome number, increases in size, and then divides to give two identical daughter cells. The doubling of the chromosomes before each division ensures that each daughter cell receives the full and identical set of chromosomes present in the original cell. The spermatogonia continue to divide rather actively during fetal life, but after birth and until the male reaches puberty, the spermatogonia seem to become quiescent.

At puberty, when the male becomes sexually mature (see Chapter 2), the continuous production of mature spermatozoa begins. Under the influence of FSH and LH the spermatogonia become transformed from round cells containing the diploid number of 46 chromosomes to tadpolelike mature sperm with a haploid number of 23 chromosomes. This maturation process is called *spermatogenesis*. To ensure a continual production of sperm, the spermatogonia again begin to proliferate by additional mitotic divisions. The descendants of those divisions are of two cellular types referred to as type A spermatogonia and type B spermatogonia. The type A cells do not themselves develop into reproductively capable sperm, but continue to reproduce by mitosis; the descendants of these divisions are more type A cells and additional type B cells. The type B cells give rise to primary spermatocytes, the cells that undergo meiosis to become mature spermatozoa capable of fertilization.

Meiosis in primary spermatocytes begins with the replication of the 46 chromosomes so that each chromosome has an exact copy of itself attached to it. The primary spermatocytes then undergo the first maturation division. The products of this division are called secondary spermatocytes. These quickly divide again to yield four haploid *spermatids*, two with 22 autosomes and an X chromosome and two with 22 autosomes and a Y chromosome. With the formation of spermatids the reduction of the diploid number of 46 chromosomes to the haploid number of 23 is complete. The remainder of sperm cell development involves the metamorphosis of predominantly round spermatids to elongated cells that have the characteristic head, midpiece, and tail portions.

During the maturation process the developing sperm cells lie adjacent to large nutrient cells, called *Sertoli cells*, that extend from the outer or basement membrane of the seminiferous tubule toward the central lumen (Figure 5–5). Spermatocytes undergoing meiosis tend to be clustered around the portion of the Sertoli cells nearest the outer membrane of the seminiferous tubule. After meiosis is completed, the haploid spermatids move toward the lumen of the tubule as they metamorphose into spermatogonia. Movement along the Sertoli cells is complete when the spermatozoa reach the tubule lumen.

Studies of spermatogenesis using the electron microscope have shown that spermatocytes progress through the various stages of the maturation process as interconnected pairs (Bloom and Fawcett, 1968). Apparently, in the last division of a type B spermatogonium, the daughter cells remain connected by an intercellular bridge. Thus, the final incomplete division of a type B spermatogonium results in a connected pair of primary spermatocytes, which after the first maturation division become four joined secondary spermatocytes. These secondary spermatocytes undergo the second maturation division to yield eight interconnected spermatids (Figure

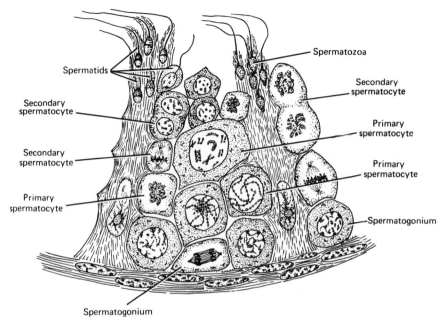

Spermatozoa

Spermatids

Secondary
spermatocyte

Secondary
spermatocyte

Primary
spermatocyte

Secondary
spermatocyte

Primary
spermatocyte

Primary
spermatocyte

Spermatogonium

Spermatogonium

FIGURE 5-5

Maturation of spermatozoa in the seminiferous tubules of the testis. From L. Arey, *Developmental Anatomy*, 8th ed. (Philadelphia: Saunders, 1974). Reprinted by permission.

5–6). The cellular bridges between the eight spermatids break down some time in the maturation process after meiosis is completed and before the cells become spermatozoa.

MATURATION OF OVA

The maturation of ova in the ovary is called *oogenesis*. Like the sperm, all mature ova arise from primordial cells—called *oogonia*—which can be found in the fetal gonadal tissue about the fifth week after fertilization. The oogonia lie embedded in a surrounding layer of cells, one oogonium and its cellular capsule being called a primordial ovarian follicle. From the fifth to about the thirty-second

101

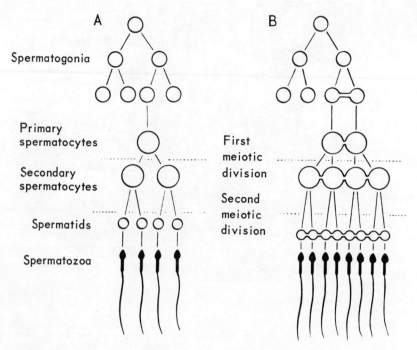

A   B

Spermatogonia

Primary
spermatocytes

First
meiotic
division

Secondary
spermatocytes

Second
meiotic
division

Spermatids

Spermatozoa

FIGURE 5-6
Spermatids with connecting intercellular bridges. From W. Bloom and D. Fawcett, *Textbook of Histology*, 7th ed. (Philadelphia: Saunders, 1967). Reprinted by permission.

week of development, the oogonia increase in number mitotically, but at the end of that period the cells gradually stop dividing and the total number of ova a woman will ever have reaches its maximum number, ranging between five and ten million.

After the cessation of mitosis all the oogonia enter the first stage of meiosis: chromosome replication and pairing. This is in contrast to meiosis in maturing sperm, which does not begin until puberty and which occurs in only a fraction of the total number of spermatogonia at one time. In this stage of their development, the developing ova are referred to as *primary oocytes,* and the ovarian follicle, consisting of the primary oocyte and a single layer of follicle cells, is called a *primary follicle.*

Although the developing ova begin meiosis while the female is still an embryo, none of them complete the process unless they are

TABLE 5.2
THE NUMBER OF GERM CELLS AND OVA AT DIFFERENT STAGES
IN HUMAN DEVELOPMENT

Fertilization age	Number present in ovary
6 weeks	600,000 (germ cells)
20 weeks	7,000,000 (oocytes)
Newborn	2,000,000 (oocytes)
7 years	500,000 (oocytes)
22 years	300,000 (oocytes)

SOURCE   A. Barnes, *Intrauterine Development* (Philadelphia: Lea and Febiger, 1968), p. 10.

ovulated and fertilized. For some primary oocytes, this may be a period of as many as 45 years.

During the course of her fertile lifetime, a woman will produce approximately 400 mature, fertilizable ova, one each month for thirty to forty years, even though she is originally endowed with five to ten million oogonia present in the ovaries during fetal life—the potential to mother the population of a large city. Gradually as a woman grows older, the number of ova decreases (Table 5–2). By birth, for example, there are about two million primary oocytes remaining in the ovaries, and at puberty, a woman is left with 300,000 to 500,000 premature ova. This is less than 10 percent of the original total. Through the succeeding years, there is a continued loss of primary oocytes in addition to the monthly ovulations until eventually there are no ova left in either ovary. This occurs in most women in the fourth or fifth decade of life.

THE MENSTRUAL CYCLE

The human female's fertility cycle, or menstrual cycle, recurs every 28 days, although this is the average or "ideal" cycle length. In actuality, menstrual cycles in most normal adult women range in length from 26 to 34 days, and longer or shorter cycles are possible. During each cycle an ovum in one of the two ovaries undergoes maturation and is ovulated sometime near the middle of the cycle. In the half of the cycle preceding ovulation, the cells of the follicle that surround the ovum proliferate, and some of them begin to secrete estrogen. After the ovum is released, the entire follicle undergoes a dramatic change to become what is called a corpus luteum. The *corpus luteum* is a major hormone secreting structure, producing both estrogen and progesterone, the latter hormone being primarily responsible for the preparation of the "estrogen-primed" uterus to accept a fertilized ovum.

After ovulation, if the ovum is fertilized and it implants in the uterus, a pregnancy begins. If the ovum is not fertilized, however, it dies within a couple of days, and the proliferated lining of the uterus and the blood vessels that supply it degenerate, and menstrual bleeding begins.

By convention, the first day of menstrual bleeding is considered to mark the beginning of the menstrual cycle. After menstruation stops, which usually occurs within four or five days after the onset of bleeding, the menstrual cycle advances into a preovulatory phase. The *preovulatory phase* of the cycle is characterized by the growth of several primary oocytes, and a proliferation of the follicle cells that surround the primary oocytes (Figure 5–7). The

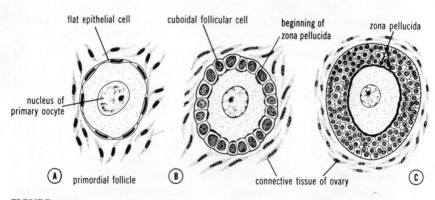

FIGURE 5-7
A. Drawing of a primordial follicle, consisting of oocyte surrounded by single layer of follicle cells. B and C. As maturation proceeds, the follicle cells grow and multiply. From J. Langman, *Medical Embryology* (Baltimore: Williams & Wilkins, 1969). Adapted from L. Shettles. Reprinted by permission.

growth of the primary oocyte and the proliferation of the follicular cells are stimulated primarily by FSH. LH is also active during this phase of the cycle, stimulating the follicle cells to secrete estrogens into the bloodstream in increasing amounts as the preovulatory phase progresses. One of the effects of the rising blood levels of estrogen is to induce the proliferation of the uterine lining from its postmenstrual basal thickness of 2 millimeters (mm) to a maximum thickness of 6 mm at midcycle.

In order to become ready for ovulation, an oocyte must complete meiosis. It should be recalled that all primary oocytes began the meiotic process during fetal life, but the process was arrested before any maturation divisions took place. In the preovulatory phase of the menstrual cycle, usually one ovum completes the first maturation division in immediate advance of its ovulation. When a primary oocyte completes the first division, the two daughter cells of the division are not of equal size. One of them receives nearly all of the cellular material present in the parent primary oocyte. This large daughter cell is referred to as a secondary oocyte, and the dwarf sister cell is called the first polar body. The secondary oocyte continues to mature, whereas the polar body degenerates. The secondary oocyte is the stage of development the ovum has reached when it is ovulated. The second maturation division to give the haploid number of chromosomes occurs only if the secondary oocyte is fertilized.

During each cycle several oocytes begin to mature. Usually, however, only one of the oocytes actually completes the maturation process to become a secondary oocyte ready for ovulation. The others are arrested at some phase in development before ovulation. These arrested oocytes degenerate, as do their surrounding follicle cells, and become scars on the ovary.

The preovulatory phase of the menstrual cycle ends near the middle of the cycle when a secondary oocyte is ovulated. By this time in the cycle the ovum has grown from a primary oocyte approximately 20 microns in diameter to a secondary oocyte with a diameter of about 140 microns. The entire follicle has undergone considerable growth as well, due to the proliferation of the follicle cells surrounding the ovum and the formation of a fluid filled cavity within the follicle called the antrum. At the time of ovulation the entire follicle, measuring perhaps 10 mm in diameter,

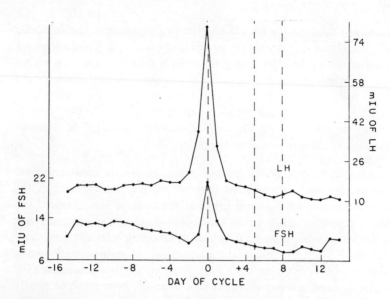

FIGURE 5-8
Levels of serum FSH and LH during the menstrual cycle. From G. Ross, *Recent Progress in Hormone Research,* 26:22, 1970. Reprinted by permission.

bulges from the surface of the ovary ready to release the secondary oocyte. Actual release of the ovum from the follicle is stimulated by the pituitary hormone, LH, the blood level of which rises sharply just before ovulation occurs (Figure 5–8).

After ovulation, the ruptured follicle becomes transformed into a yellowish body called a corpus luteum, which, under the influence of LH, secretes both estrogen and progesterone.

If the secondary oocyte is not fertilized within two days after ovulation, it will degenerate, and fertilization during that particular menstrual cycle will not be possible. In that event, the corpus luteum ceases its production of progesterone and estrogen, some time around the twenty-fifth day of a 28-day cycle. This causes the blood levels of the sex steroids to drop dramatically, and without the stimulatory effects of these hormones, the proliferated lining of the uterus breaks up and is subsequently lost in a menstrual discharge. The lost menstruate consists of tissue debris and blood associated with the decomposition of the uterine tissue built up in the previous monthly cycle. Women lose on the average of 30 to 100 cc of blood during each menstrual period, with the heaviest bleeding occurring in the first two to three days and decreasing thereafter. Menstrual bleeding usually ends within five days after it begins, but menstrual flow lasting up to seven days is not uncommon.

If fertilization does occur, however, then the corpus luteum is maintained in a functional state beyond its normal lifetime and continues to secrete estrogens and progesterone during the first weeks of the ensuing pregnancy.

The 28-day cyclicity of the menstrual cycle is maintained by a system of hormonal regulations which ultimatly controls the amounts of FSH and LH to be secreted by the pituitary gland. As these two hormones are central to all ovulatory phenomena, having both trophic effects on the ovarian follicle and inducing the secretion of ovarian steroid hormones, their regulation is the key to controlling the entire menstrual cycle. It has already been pointed out that pituitary release of FSH and LH is stimulated by releasing factors from the brain. These agents are not the sole modifiers of FSH and LH secretion, however. Even before the discovery of releasing factors, it was known that steroid sex hormones, principally estrogens, were capable of reducing the pituitary output of FSH and LH. For example, it was known that if a female mammal had her ovaries removed, thus removing the body's major sources of sex steroid hormones, the blood levels of FSH and LH would rise. When replacement injections of estrogen were given to this animal, the blood levels of those pituitary hormones would fall. Progesterone would affect pituitary secretion of FSH and LH in the same way. Thus, the regulation of the pituitary release of FSH and LH is controlled by both releasing factors from the hypothalamus and ovarian steroid hormones, the releasing factors promoting release of the pituitary hormones and the steroid hormones inhibiting the release of pituitary hormones.

During the various phases of the menstrual cycle the gonadotropic hormones, particularly LH, stimulate the ovary to secrete steroid hormones, either estrogens in the preovulatory phase or estrogens and progesterone in the postovulatory phase. When the blood levels of these steroids rise to a certain point, they begin to inhibit the secretion of FSH and LH, probably by acting on the hypothalamus to inhibit the secretion of releasing factors. This creates an internal negative feedback loop in which the effect of releasing factors and gonadotropin secretion—the release of sex steroids into the blood—has a regulating effect on the output of the releasing factors and hence the blood level of pituitary hormones (Figure 5–9).

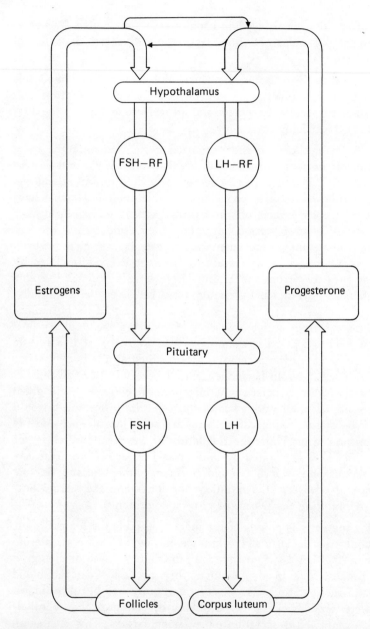

FIGURE 5-9
The regulation of the menstrual cycle by oscillations in the serum levels of hormones. Ovarian hormones modulate the hypothalamo-pituitary output of gonadotropic hormones.

MENSTRUAL DISORDERS

For some women, menstruation can be an unpleasant experience apart from the monthly inconvenience that it may bring, for it can also be a time of physical and emotional discomfort. Menstrual disorders usually appear either during the few days preceding menstrual flow or during the first two days after the onset of bleeding. Some common symptoms of menstrual troubles are abdominal cramps, backache, headache, nausea, irritability, mood swings, tension, and depression.

The most common menstrual problem is dysmenorrhea, or menstrual cramps, which is severe abdominal pain during the first few days of menstrual flow. Dysmenorrhea is most prevalent in adolescent girls, although its frequency in adult women is strikingly high. It is estimated that between 20 and 70 percent of the women suffer from menstrual cramps (Santamaria, 1969). The causes of dysmenorrhea are still debated among gynecologists, but many suggestions implicate physical defects which bring difficulty in passing the menstruate from the body. These include cervical obstruction, a small uterus, and a faulty posture associated with a sedentary occupation. There may also be psychological factors involved in the occurrence of dysmenorrhea. For example, it is felt that a negative attitude toward menstruation acquired from the parents before a girl's first menstrual period can contribute to incidence of pain at menstruation. To date none of these suggestions has been shown to be the single causative factor in all cases of dysmenorrhea. It is likely that more than one cause exists. Perhaps a combination of physical and psychological factors is involved.

Medical treatment of dysmenorrhea often involves the administration of pain-relieving drugs, sometimes in combination with psychoactive compounds to relieve depression or anxiety. Many women who experience dysmenorrhea find the severity of menstrual cramps reduced after they begin to take contraceptive pills. Although there is no firm indication that irregular hormone levels are involved in dysmenorrhea, the relief offered by the synthetic estrogens and progestogens in oral contraceptives suggests a hormonal etiology. On the other hand, the relief of dysmenorrhea might be due to the suppression of ovulation—one mode of action of the pills.

Another common menstrual problem is the so-called premenstrual syndrome, which occurs a few days before the onset of menstrual flow. The premenstrual syndrome is sometimes referred to as premenstrual tension because of the overt psychological agitation and/or depression which occurs at that time. A common physical symptom of the premenstrual syndrome is a swelling of the pelvic area due to the retention of water. This swelling can lead to transitory weight gain and a feeling of bloatedness, and it may aggravate other premenstrual problems such as nausea, backache, and general tension. Some studies have revealed that, at least for some women, the premenstrual phase of the menstrual cycle may bring an increase in the general level of sexual arousal (Masters and Johnson, 1970; Sherfey, 1966). Such heightened levels of sexual tension may be caused by the swelling in the pelvic area which mimics the physiological response to sexual stimulation. Alternatively, it may be due to the knowledge that conception is highly improbable during menstruation.

For the woman who experiences menstrual discomfort regularly, the problem may have immense significance, for its recurrence every month may adversely affect her personal life. Studies have shown that the incidence of accidents, suicides, and acute psychological distress is greater during the menstrual period than at other times of the cycle (Dalton, 1964; Pasnau, 1969). In a survey of women prisoners in England, it was found that 49 percent of 156 newly admitted prisoners had committed their crimes in the menstrual phase of the cycle (Dalton, 1964).

FERTILIZATION

With the maturation of sperm in the testes and the maturation of an ovum in an ovary and its release from the ovary at ovulation, the stage is set for fertilization to take place. During sexual intercourse when the man ejaculates, semen containing 300 to 500 million sperm is deposited in the vagina, collecting in a pool at the back of the vagina near the cervix if the woman is in the supine position. From the placement in the vagina the sperm must move through the cervix and body of the uterus and into the uterine tubes (Figure 5–10). Once the sperm enter a tube that contains a fertilizable secondary oocyte, the fusion of a single spermatozoon and the oocyte to form a zygote becomes possible.

The movement of sperm through the cervix is the first part of the journey to the uterine tubes. Normally the cervix is bathed in a mucus that is produced by crypts in the cervical walls. This mucus is usually quite viscous, and many sperm may become trapped in it. Near the time of ovulation, however, the cervical mucus becomes less viscous and therefore more lenient to the passage of sperm than at other times of the menstrual cycle. The mucus may also be beneficial to sperm transport and survival at this time of the cycle. The change in cervical mucus viscosity is due to the actions of estrogens on the cells of the cervix which produce the mucus. The rise in estrogen levels to a midcycle maximum coordinates the change in cervical mucus viscosity with ovulation. Thus, as the ovum is freed from the ovary at midcycle, the "cervical barrier" is relaxed in order to facilitate the transport of sperm into the uterus.

Sperm that traverse the cervix enter the body of the uterus and are transported toward the uterine tubes with the aid of muscular contractions of the uterus. Uterine contractions that enhance sperm transport can be caused by several stimuli. For example, contractions of the uterus occur when a woman experiences orgasm. It is also known that semen contains biochemical substances called prostaglandins which, when given to a woman either intravenously or inserted in the vagina, are capable of inducing uterine contractions. It is not yet certain whether prostaglandins introduced into the vagina during sexual intercourse cause uterine contractions capable of assisting sperm transport to the uterine tubes. Another possible stimulus of uterine contractions is a hormone from the posterior pituitary gland called oxytocin. The blood levels of oxytocin have been shown to rise in women during and after sexual intercourse, and it is known that oxytocin can stimulate contractions of the uterus.

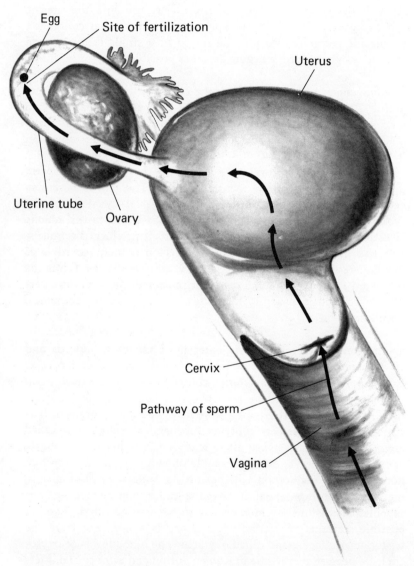

FIGURE 5-10
Pathway of spermatozoa from the vagina to the uterine tubes.

After sperm have moved through the uterus, they arrive at the entrances of the pair of uterine tubes or oviducts. Each tube is connected to the uterus by a narrow uterotubal junction. Because of the narrow diameter of the uterotubal junction, many sperm never enter either of the tubes. This has the effect of reducing the number of sperm available to take part in fertilization. And since only one of the tubes contains an ovum, the sperm that enter the "empty tube" have no chance to unite with it.

Although normal ejaculates may contain as many as 500 million sperm, only a small fraction of that number ever reach the site of fertilization in one of the uterine tubes. The great majority of sperm either never succeed in negotiating barriers to their migration—the cervix and uterotubal junctions—or are ingested by white blood cells which infiltrate the lining of the uterus and tubes.

Sperm that manage to get into the oviducts become transported toward the ovarian end of the tube principally by muscular contractions of the tube and also by the fact that they tend to swim oriented against the beat of the tubal cilia, which is directed toward the uterine end of the tube. If an ovum is in the tube, having been captured by the oviductal fimbriae after ovulation, it and its 3000 or so attached follicle cells are transported toward the uterus by the action of the tubal cilia. Thus, the gametes are simultaneously propelled in opposite directions while inside the tube. The actual meeting of one or more spermatozoa and the ovum is apparently caused by this movement of the gametes toward each other.

The actual fusion of a spermatozoon and an ovum first requires the removal of the follicle cells from the circumference of the ovum, a final stage of maturation of the sperm while inside the uterus and oviducts, called *capacitation*, and then penetration of the zona pellucida. The follicular cells that surround the ovum become dispersed when exposed to tubal fluids and due to the mechanical action of the tubes. Capacitation of sperm is a function of a factor (or factors) present in the tubal fluids. Sperm taken from male animals are not capable of fertilization unless they are first exposed to tubal fluids. Penetration of the zona pellucida by sperm is accomplished by the enzymatic degradation of its gelatinous substance.

Several sperm may take part in the destruction of the zona pellucida; however, only one succeeds in uniting with the ovum (Figure 5–11). The fertilizing spermatozoon contacts the ovum and its

113

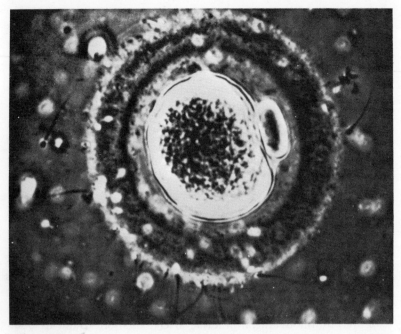

FIGURE 5-11

Fertilization of human ovum. Spermatozoa surround the ovum and attached cumulus cells. Many spermatozoa make contact with the ovum but only one succeeds in penetrating the ovum's outer membranes to effect fertilization. From L. Shettles, *Ovum Hamanum* (New York: Haffner, 1960). Reprinted by permission.

membrane fuses with the membrane of the ovum. The head and tail portions of the spermatozoon then enter the ovum, and the spermatozoon nucleus (located in the head portion) enlarges to become what is called the male pronucleus. The fusion of the sperm and the ovum stimulates the ovum's second meiotic division which, like the first meiotic division, produces one daughter cell with most of the cellular material and a small nonfunctional cell referred to as the second polar body. The large daughter cell is called female pronucleus. The fertilized ovum, then, consists of the pair of pronuclei.

After the fertilizing sperm has made contact and fused with the ovum, a mechanism which blocks the entry of additional sperm is activated. Before fertilization, a layer of granules underlies the ovum's membrane, and after penetration of the ovum's membrane by a spermatozoon, these granules break down and disappear. It is thought that the breakdown of these granules affords the block to polyspermy.

INFERTILITY

If a couple is unable to produce a baby after attempting to do so over a reasonable period of time, then they are considered to be infertile. Infertility occurs in approximately 10 to 15 percent of American couples; it can be caused by a host of physiological and anatomical deficiencies in either the male or the female reproductive systems which can make successful fertilization improbable or impossible, or render the female unable to carry a pregnancy to term (Table 5–3).

Many times the causes of infertility in a husband or wife can be diagnosed and treated successfully so that the formerly infertile couple will be able to have children. For example, when either nutritional deficiencies, fatigue, excessive smoking, drinking, or drug taking are the cause of infertility, the ability to have children can be restored by a change in living habits. It is also possible to correct causes of infertility resulting from physical defects in the reproductive organs by employing corrective surgery. And inadequate hormone secretion can usually be treated by giving replacement therapy with natural hormones, synthetic hormones, and certain fertility drugs such as clomiphene citrate.

Infertility in the male is often the result of the man's inability to produce or deposit in the vagina normal numbers of healthy sperm. For example, a man is infertile if he produces too few sperm, *oligospermia*, or no sperm at all, *azospermia*. Sometimes the number of sperm produced is adequate, but for some reason a high proportion of them are abnormal in shape and therefore cannot take part in fertilization. Infertility may also be caused by a man not producing an adequate volume of seminal fluid. Sometimes it is not the production of normal amounts of sperm that is the infertility problem, but rather the inability to deposit the sperm in the vagina. If a man cannot achieve or maintain an erection, he is usually incapable of insemination and hence fertilization is impossible.

TABLE 5.3
ETIOLOGICAL INTERPRETATION OF CAUSE OF INFERTILITY AS
RELATED TO HUSBAND, WIFE, AND THE COUPLE AS A UNIT

Female factors	Male factors
General	*General*
Dietary disturbances	Fatigue
Severe anemias	Excess smoking, alcohol
Anxiety, fear, etc.	Excess coitus
(hypothalamus)	Fear, impotence, etc.
Developmental	*Developmental*
Uterine absence, hypoplasia	Undescended testis
Uterine anomalies	Testicular germinal aplasia
Gonadal dysgenesis	Hypospadias
	Klinefelter's syndrome
Endocrine	
Pituitary failure	*Endocrine*
Thyroid disturbances	Pituitary failure
Adrenal hyperplasia	Thyroid deficiency
Ovarian failure, polycystic disease	Adrenal hyperplasia
Genital Disease	*Genital Disease*
Pelvic-inflammation, tuberculosis	Orchitis, mumps
Tubal obstructions	Venereal disease
Endometriosis	Prostatitis
Myomata and polyps	
Cervicitis	
Vaginitis	

Male-female factors

Marital maladjustments
Sex problems
Ignorance (timing, douching, sperm
   leakage, etc.)
Low fertility index
Immunologic incompatibility

SOURCE S. J. Behrman and R. W. Kistner, *Progress in Infertility* (Boston:
Little, Brown, 1968), p. 6.

When the cause of a couple's infertility is diagnosed as the husband's inability to produce normal healthy sperm in sufficient number to effect fertilization, it is still possible for that couple to have children if the wife is artificially inseminated. *Artificial insemination* is the process whereby sperm are introduced into the woman's vagina or uterus by a doctor. Thus, in the case where the husband's sperm count is low, and infertility is therefore due to the fact that a sufficient number of sperm cannot reach the uterine tubes after sexual intercourse, artificial insemination with the husband's sperm will give the sperm a "head start" by placing them inside the female reproductive tract beyond vaginal and cervical barriers to sperm transport. If infertility is caused by the fact that the husband cannot produce any normal sperm, artificial insemination is possible with the sperm of a donor.

The technique of artificial insemination has been used successfully in the breeding of farm animals for many years. In cattle breeding, for example, the semen of a prize bull can be used to inseminate many cows who are perhaps hundreds or thousands of miles from the bull. The semen of the bull is frozen in a special way and shipped to breeders who artificially inseminate the cows. In recent years there has been an interest in developing techniques to freeze human semen with the ultimate goal of using it at some later time. This would permit the storing of donor semen (so-called *"cryo-banking"*) for use at appropriate times. One possible use of the cryo-banking of semen would be in family planning. A man could have several semen specimens frozen and then have a vasectomy, a method of birth control that prevents the movement of sperm from the epididymis to the urethra (see Chapter 8). Then, when the couple wanted to have a child, the wife could be artificially inseminated with her husband's semen, taken from the storage bank.

The causes of infertility in women usually involve problems in the transport of sperm from the vagina to the uterine tubes. For example, it is estimated that nearly 20 percent of female infertility cases are due to cervical obstruction alone (Taymore, 1969). Such cervical obstructions can be either anatomical deformities of the cervix or the production of cervical mucus hostile to sperm survival. In either case, the sperm are prevented from entering the uterus and completing the rendezvous with the ovum. Other factors that can impede or prevent sperm transport in the female reproductive tract are malformations of the uterus, constriction of one or both of the uterine tubes, and the existence of an environment hostile to sperm in the uterus or uterine tubes. This latter defect is often caused by improper hormonal regulation of the physiology of these organs.

One theoretical treatment of infertility caused by difficulties in sperm transport within the female reproductive tract is to begin the fertilization process outside the female's body. Then, once the ovum is fertilized, it can be placed inside the uterus where it can develop. Such a process of *in vitro* fertilization has been successfully carried out in laboratory animals and with a few human ova. The procedure involves removing a mature ovum from the ovary of the female and placing it in a supportive culture medium in a test tube or dish. Then sperm are taken from a male and placed in the culture medium with the ovum, a drop of fluid from a uterine tube is added to effect capacitation of the sperm, and then fertilization is allowed to take place. If a couple's infertility problem is due to the fact that sperm are not able to travel successfully from the vagina to the uterine tubes, this type of medical intervention, if perfected, could overcome the problem.

Other difficulties encountered with sperm transport relate to the environment provided the migrating sperm by the vagina, uterus, and uterine tubes. It is believed that the secretions of these organs have important maintenance functions with regard to sperm survival. Thus, if these secretions are not present in sufficient amounts, or if their composition is not correct, then sperm may be prohibited from continuing their migration. The maintenance of many of the conditions supportive of sperm transport in the female is a function of the ovarian steroid hormones, estrogen and progesterone. Hence the undersecretion of these hormones from the maturing follicle or the corpus luteum may be the direct cause of female infertility. And since steroid production by the ovary is dependent upon adequate stimulatory effects of pituitary hormones, FSH and LH, subnormal amounts of these hormones may cause infertility as well. The undersecretion of pituitary hormones may also make a woman unable to ovulate. In either of these hormone deficiencies, replacement therapy with exogenous hormones may restore fertility.

Sometimes the cause of infertility is associated with the time of coitus. For fertilization to occur, sperm must be present in the uterine tube while a fertilizable ovum is there also. Since an ovum is viable for only a day or two after ovulation, this means that intercourse and insemination must take place at, or very near, the time of ovulation. Sperm in the female reproductive tract at any other time in the menstrual cycle are, of course, nonreproductive.

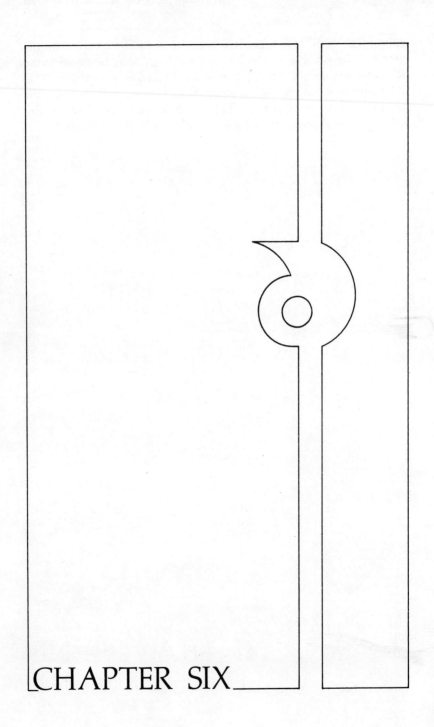

CHAPTER SIX

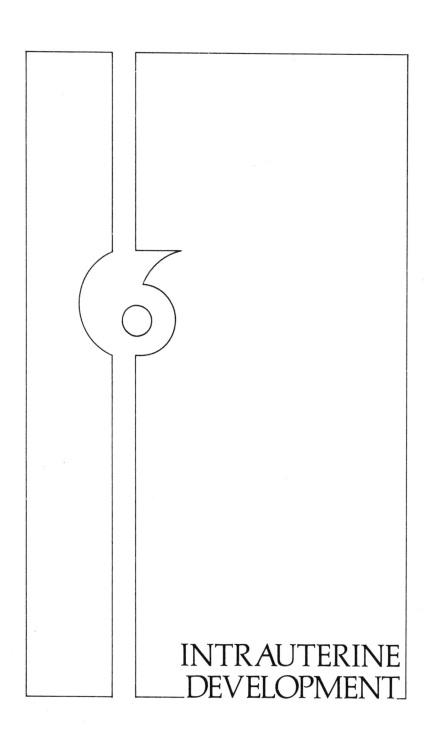

INTRAUTERINE DEVELOPMENT

With the fusion of a spermatozoon and an ovum at fertilization, the phase of the human life cycle devoted to the intrauterine development of a fetus begins. During this phase of life a multitude of new cells arises by means of successive mitotic divisions of the single-celled zygote formed at fertilization. And as the new cells form, they differentiate into the many specialized cells that make up the various tissues and organs of the human body. The period of intrauterine development ends approximately 266 days after fertilization when the fetus is expelled from the mother's body at birth.

The divisions of the zygote begin within 24 to 30 hours after fertilization when the zygote divides into two cells called *blastomeres* (Figure 6–1). The two original blastomeres each divide again to yield four cells, the four cells divide to become eight, and so on. The first few divisions take place at about daily intervals, so that within three days after fertilization the conceptus is a relatively compact ball of about 12 to 16 cells called a *morula,* which is the Latin word for mulberry.

Since most of fetal development takes place in the uterus but fertilization occurs in the uterine tube, the conceptus moves from the uterine tube to the uterus within the first four days after fertilization (Figure 6–2). The journey through the uterine tube from the site of fertilization to the uterus takes place while the first few cell divisions are occurring. By the time of the formation of the morula, the conceptus has completed its tubal migration and is near the uterotubal junction.

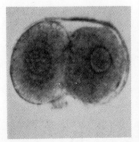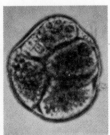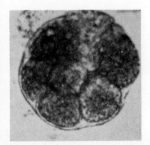

FIGURE 6-1
Development of human zygote from the two-cell stage to late morula. By courtesy of the Carnegie Institution of Washington.

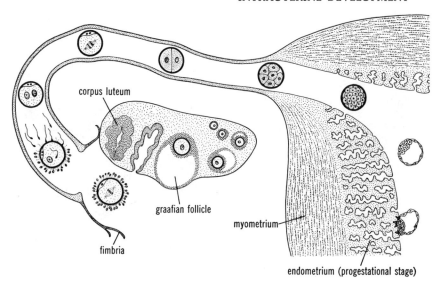

FIGURE 6-2

Movement of the conceptus from the site of fertilization in the uterine tube to the uterus. The two-cell stage occurs approximately 30 hours after fertilization. The conceptus enters the uterus as a morula approximately 4 days after fertilization. Implantation begins approximately 6 days after fertilization. From J. Langman, *Medical Embryology* (Baltimore: Williams & Wilkins, 1969). Reprinted by permission.

The entrance of the conceptus into the cavity of the uterus is believed to occur near the fourth day of development. By this time the conceptus, now referred to as a *blastocyst,* is comprised of between 50 and 100 cells that surround a fluid-filled cavity called a blastocoel. An actual 4-day-old human blastocyst (recovered from a woman's uterus after surgery) was found to consist of 58 cells. Fifty-three of the cells circumscribed the blastocyst and were called the *trophoblast,* and 5 of the cells were concentrated at one pole of the blastocyst and referred to as the *inner cell mass.* Another specimen, believed to be 4½ days old, has also been recovered. It was found to consist of 107 cells, 99 making up the trophoblast and 8 contributing to the inner cell mass. The cells of the trophoblast give rise to the fetal portion of the placenta, and the inner cell mass develops into the fetal body (Figure 6–3).

Within two or three days after its arrival in the uterus, the blastocyst attaches to the uterine lining, usually near the midportion

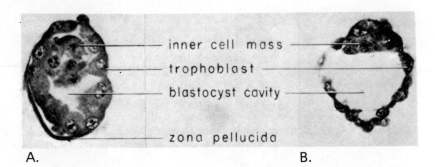

inner cell mass

trophoblast

blastocyst cavity

zona pellucida

A.   B.

FIGURE 6-3
A. 4-day-old human blastocyst consisting of 58 cells. B. 4½-day-old human blastocyst consisting of 107 cells. By courtesy of the Carnegie Institution of Washington.

of the posterior uterine wall. Soon after the blastocyst attaches to the uterus, the trophoblast begins to invade the uterine lining. This is the beginning of the *implantation process.* The invasion of the uterine lining by advancing trophoblast continues for about one or two days, and on about the ninth day after fertilization, the blastocyst is almost completely embedded in the uterus (Figure 6–4). By the eleventh or twelfth day, implantation of the blastocyst is complete and the uterine lining grows over the implanted blastocyst until only a small bulge is visible on the inner surface of the uterus.

Development of the fetal body begins during the second week after fertilization when the inner cell mass differentiates into a flattened disc consisting of two layers of cells applied to one another. One of these cell layers is called the *ectoderm* and the other is called the *entoderm.* During the third week of development a third layer of cells arises between the original ectodermal-entodermal bilayer. This third layer of cells is called the *mesoderm.*

The ectoderm, the entoderm, and the mesoderm are referred to as germ layers, for they give rise to all of the specialized cells that make up the human body (Table 6–1). The ectoderm differentiates into the central nervous system, the peripheral nervous system, and the sensory epithelium of the sense organs. It also gives rise to the epidermis including hair, nails, and subcutaneous glands; the pituitary; the enamel layer of teeth; and the linings of other body organs. The mesoderm gives rise to connective tissue,

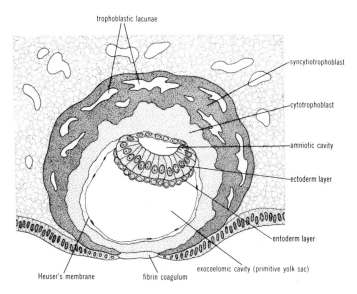

trophoblastic lacunae

syncytiotrophoblast

cytotrophoblast

amniotic cavity

ectoderm layer

entoderm layer

exocoelomic cavity (primitive yolk sac)

fibrin coagulum

Heuser's membrane

FIGURE 6-4
Drawing of a 9-day-old human blastocyst, showing ectoderm and entoderm layers. From J. Langman, *Medical Embryology* (Baltimore: Williams & Wilkins, 1969). Reprinted by permission.

cartilage and bone; striated and smooth muscle; blood and lymph cells, and the walls of the heart, blood, and lymph vessels; the kidneys, the gonads and their corresponding ducts; part of the adrenal gland; and the spleen. The entoderm contributes to the epithelial lining of the digestive tract, the urinary bladder and urethra, the Eustachian tube, tympanic cavity, and the respiratory tract. It also gives rise to part of the tonsils, thyroid and parathyroid glands, the thymus, liver, and pancreas.

The differentiation of the ectoderm, mesoderm, and entoderm into the various tissues and organs of the body takes place mostly during the fourth to eighth weeks of development. During this time the major organ systems of the body are established.

Central Nervous System   The central nervous system originates as an open-ended tube formed during the third week of development. The ends of the tube become closed off during the fourth week, and the anterior end of the closed tube then differentiates into the brain and the posterior portion becomes the spinal cord.

125

TABLE 6.1
THE GERM-LAYER ORIGIN OF HUMAN TISSUES

Ectoderm	Mesoderm (including mesenchyme)	Entoderm
Epidermis, including:	Muscle (all types)	Epithelium of:
Cutaneous glands.	Connective tissue;	Pharynx, including:
Hair: nails; lens.	cartilage; bone;	Root of tongue.
Epithelium of:	notochord.	Auditory tube, etc.
Sense organs.	Blood; bone marrow.	Tonsils; thyroid.
Nasal cavity;	Lymphoid tissue.	Parathyroids;
sinuses.	Epithelium of:	thymus.
Mouth, including:	Blood vessels;	Larynx; trachea; lungs.
Oral glands;	lymphatics.	Digestive tube,
enamel.	Body cavities.	including:
Anal canal.	Kidney; ureter.	Associated glands.
Nervous tissue,	Gonads; genital	Bladder.
including:	ducts.	Vagina (all?);
Hypophysis.	Suprarenal cortex.	vestibule.
Chromaffin tissue.	Joint cavities, etc.	Urethra, including:
		Associated glands

SOURCE   L. B. Arey, *Developmental Anatomy* (Philadelphia: Saunders, 1965), p. 83.

Respiratory System   During the third week a primitive respiratory tract develops from the tubelike foregut. Eventually a membrane forms that separates the primitive respiratory tract from the digestive tube, except in the region of the larynx. During the fourth week the trachea forms out of the respiratory tube with two lateral outpocketings which are called lung buds. The lug buds soon branch into main bronchi, which then branch and rebranch into the complete bronchial tree.

Digestive System   The intestinal tract develops as a tube during the fourth week. It eventually elongates and undergoes torsion to form the permanent digestive tract: esophagus, stomach, duodenum, small and large bowel, and rectum. Outpocketings of the digestive tube form the liver, gall bladder, and pancreas.

Cardiovascular System   By the third week of development the heart forms as a straight tube, and it begins to beat about a week later. By the sixth week the heart has developed the four-chambered adult form. As organs develop, blood vessels develop within them, and blood cells form in the blood vessels themselves, the liver, spleen, and bone marrow.

Reproductive System   The gonadal ridges are formed by the fourth week after fertilization, and during the fifth week the germ cells migrate from the yolk sac to the as yet undifferentiated gonads. By the eighth week the testes or ovaries have differentiated. The genital duct systems then begin to form (see Chapter 2).

Urinary System   Three pairs of excretory systems unfold sequentially during development. The first excretory system, called the pronephros, eventually degenerates. The second system is called the mesonephros. It eventually differentiates into the male genital ducts or degenerates in the female. The permanent kidneys in both sexes develop from a third fetal excretory system called the metanephros, which forms the many millions of excretory units that comprise the adult kidney. The collecting system of tubules that is also part of the permanent kidney forms from outpocketings of the mesonephros called ureteric buds.

By the end of the eighth week of development most of the body's organs have achieved their permanent form and the fetus' external appearance is unquestionably human (Figure 6–5). The head is completely developed, although it is larger in proportion to the rest of the body than at later times in life. Eyes, ears, nose, and mouth are present on the face. The arms and legs have developed and have a full complement of fingers and toes. At this stage of development the fetus weighs about 1 gram and is about 2 or 3 cm long. During the remainder of the period of intrauterine development the fetus grows considerably and at birth weighs about 3000 grams and is approximately 50 cm in head-to-heel length.

Fetal development and growth takes place with the fetus enclosed in a fluid-filled membranous sac called the *amnion*. The amnion forms from the trophoblast during the second week of development and eventually completely surrounds the fetus, separating the fetus from contact with the walls of the uterine cavity. Throughout the period of intrauterine development the fetus is surrounded by the amnion and the fluid it contains (Figure 6–6). By develop-

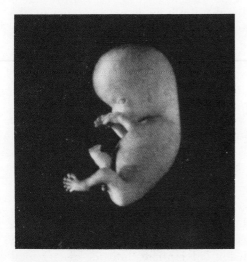

FIGURE 6-5
A 9-week-old human embryo. Courtesy of the Carnegie Institution of Washington.

ing in this aqueous environment, the fetus is able to grow unencumbered by the mother's internal organs. The amniotic fluid also protects the fetus from experiencing possibly damaging jolts when the mother changes her body position. At birth, the amnion ruptures before the fetus emerges from the uterus, an event sometimes referred to as "the breaking of the bag of water."

Understanding the mechanisms which control the development of the many specialized cells that comprise the permanent body organs from the zygote and the seemingly identical blastomeres is one of the most challenging areas of investigation in modern biology. Since all cells contain identical genetic information encoded in the DNA of the 46 chromosomes, the formation of a specialized cell type is the result of controlled and selected gene expression. If the same genes were expressed in every cell, all cells would be identical. In order to produce a given specialized cell type, the activities of some of the genes in a differentiating cell are repressed whereas others are expressed to form and maintain the cell in a specialized state.

Experiments with various animal embryos indicate that the differentiation of the cells of a particular tissue or organ can be stimulated by the presence of a neighboring tissue or chemical product

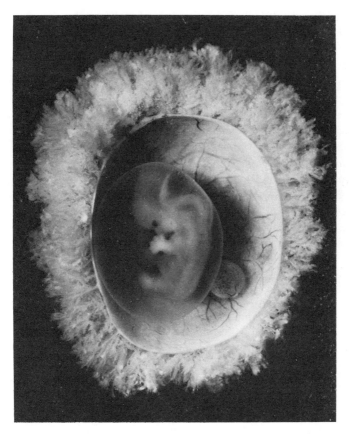

FIGURE 6-6
Human fetus surrounded by amnion and amniotic fluid. By courtesy of the
Carnegie Institution of Washington.

such as a hormone. It is known, for example, that the ureteric
bud, an outgrowth of the mesonephros, stimulates the formation
of permanent kidney tubules from metanephrogenic tissue. If the
ureteric bud is experimentally removed from the locale of the metanephrogenic tissue destined to become kidney tubules, the tubules
fail to differentiate. The ureteric bud is said to be the "inductor"
of kidney tubules. Other examples of tissue induction include the
formation of the lens of the eye from precursor ectodermal tissue
induced by the neighboring optic vesicle, and the induction of
male genitalia from primitive genital organs by the influence of
androgenic hormones secreted by the fetal testis.

129

The mechanism by which the ureteric bud induces the differentiation of metanephrogenic tissue into kidney tubules has been studied using tissue culture techniques (Grobstein, 1959). Metanephrogenic tissue destined to differentiate into kidney tubules was removed from mouse embryos before differentiation occurred and was placed in a tissue culture medium. Removed from the embryo, this tissue failed to differentiate. If the metanephrogenic tissue was placed in the same culture medium with tissue from the ureteric bud, however, kidney tubules formed as in the intact mouse embryo. In a variation of this experiment, a porous filter was placed between the metanephrogenic tissue and the tissue of the ureteric bud so that contact beween the two tissues was prevented. Even with the porous filter between the two tissues the ureteric bud was able to induce the differentiation of kidney tubules from the metanephrogenic tissue. It was concluded that the induction of kidney tubules by ureteric bud tissue was mediated by the transfer of a molecule or molecules through the filter which in some way induced the formation of kidney tubules.

From these and other similar experiments it is thought that the differentiation of a particular specialized cell type from a precursor cell is induced by chemical substances produced in neighboring cells, probably of a different type. This suggests that the unfolding of a fetal body from the zygote is controlled by a cascade of biochemical signals. The first cells produce inductor substances that induce the differentiation of newly formed cells, which themselves may produce additional inductor substances which induce the differentiation of additional cell types and so on until the entire body is differentiated.

THE PLACENTA AND FETAL CIRCULATION

Fetal development requires certain materials for growth and the maintenance of life-sustaining physiological processes. Primary among these substances is food, which is needed to supply energy for metabolic work and to provide the building blocks of the body's tissues and organs. In addition to food, a supply of molecular oxygen must be available so food can be converted to energy efficiently. The developing embryo must also have an adequate supply of vitamins and minerals to participate in the many biochemical reactions which sustain life.

The ultimate source of these life-sustaining and growth materials is the fetus' environment. Embryos of most aquatic animals develop in open water, for example, and they obtain their life support substances by direct diffusion with the surrounding aqueous environment. The shelled embryos of reptiles and birds derive their nutrient from a large supply of yolk enclosed in the egg with them, and oxygen enters through the porous eggshell. All mammalian embryos (except the monotremes whose embryos develop inside eggs) develop inside the uterus of their mother, which affords them protection from environmental hazards such as predators and bad weather, but at the same time removes them from direct contact with the external environment. In order to survive and grow inside the uterus, they must have some way to acquire necessary materials from their surroundings. This is accomplished by the establishment of a supportive relationship between the embryo and the mother whereby the embryo derives its needed materials from the mother's body. While developing in the uterus, the fetus carries out exchange with the environment by using the maternal bloodstream to bring it food, oxygen, and other substances and to carry away waste products. Thus the mother's body is an intermediary in the exchange of materials between the fetus and the external environment.

The fetal-maternal supportive relationship is maintained by the *placenta*, a specialized organ that consists of tissues contributed by both the fetus and the mother. In humans, the placenta forms mainly from the trophoblast after the blastocyst has implanted in the uterus. The trophoblast invades the lining of the uterus, advancing in fingerlike projections called *chorionic villi*. As the villi push into the surrounding uterine lining small spaces appear in the trophoblast between the villi. These spaces are called lacunae or primitive intervillous spaces (Figure 6–7). Eventually the tips of the advancing chorionic villi come upon maternal blood vessels. The walls of these blood vessels are broken down and maternal blood enters the lacunae. This takes place about 11 or 12 days

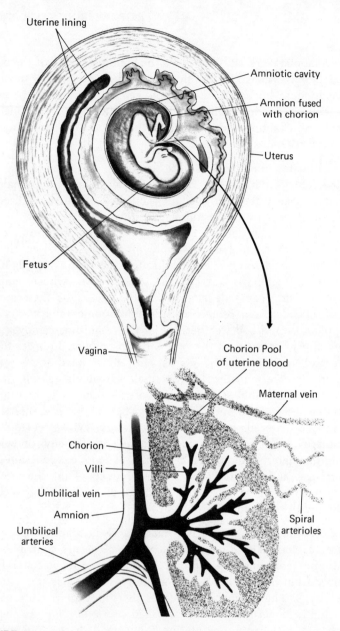

Uterine lining

Amniotic cavity

Amnion fused with chorion

Uterus

Fetus

Vagina

Chorion Pool of uterine blood

Maternal vein

Chorion

Villi

Umbilical vein

Amnion

Umbilical arteries

Spiral arterioles

FIGURE 6-7

Placental blood flow. Maternal blood arrives at the placental site via uterine arteries which then terminate in maternal blood sinusoids. Fetal blood flows through the umbilical arteries, through capillaries in the chorionic villi, and then back to the fetus through the umbilical vein. At no time do the two bloodstreams mix. Nutrients and waste products are exchanged across placental tissue.

after fertilization. The blood-filled lacunae ultimately coalesce to form a unified pool of maternal blood, and many new villi, formed by the branching and rebranching of previously formed villi, grow into the blood-filled space. By the third week of development, blood vessels form in the chorionic villi which, after the formation of fetal blood elements and the fetal heart, begin to carry blood from the fetus to the chorionic villi and back to the fetus. The exchange of nutrients and waste products takes place by the diffusion and active transport of materials from maternal blood occupying the intervillous space across tissue of the chorionic villi and into the blood supply of the fetus that flows through the blood vessels of the chorionic villi. At no time do the bloodstreams of fetus and mother actually mix; fetal blood flow is from the fetal body to the chorionic villi and back to the fetus, and maternal blood flow is from the mother's heart to the intervillous space of the placenta and back to the heart.

The flow of blood from the body of the fetus and from the placenta is through the umbilical cord, which contains three blood vessels— two arteries and one vein. Beginning at the fetal heart, blood is pumped through the umbilical arteries to the chorionic villi of the placenta where the exchange with maternal blood in the inter-villous space occurs. The venous capillaries of the villi that carry the material away from the exchange site eventually merge into the umbilical vein. Once in the umbilical vein the oxygen-rich, nutritious blood flows back to the fetal heart, which pumps it throughout the fetal body.

Blood circulation in the fetus is different from that in the adult because of the unique placental relationship. With fetal supplies of oxygen coming from the placenta instead of the lungs, blood flow to the lungs to pick up oxygen does not occur. Thus, in the fetus, much of the blood that would flow to the lungs if the fetus were to breathe air is diverted through structures in the circulatory system that are present only during fetal life.

One of the structures that help divert blood flow away from the lungs consists of a hole in the inner wall of the heart that separates the right and left atria. This hole is called the *foramen ovale*, and it allows some of the blood which enters the right atrium to flow directly into the left atrium without first passing through the pul-monary circulation as it does in the adult; namely, right ventricle

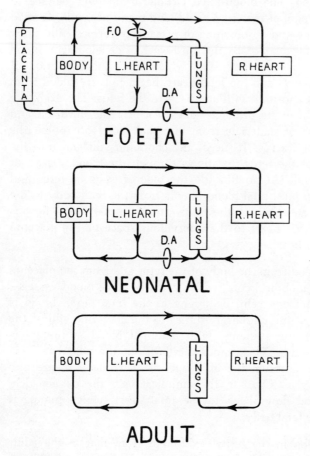

FIGURE 6-8

Comparison of circulatory systems in fetus, neonate, and adult. (F.D. is the foramen orale and D.A. is the ductus arteriosus.) From G. V. Born, *Symp. Quant. Biol.*, 19:106 (1954). Reprinted by permission.

→ pulmonary arteries → lung → pulmonary veins → left atrium. This segment of the entering bloodstream travels directly through the foramen ovale to the left atrium, on into the left ventricle, and then out of the heart into the aorta (Figure 6–8). The blood that is not shunted through the foramen ovale passes through the right atrium to the right ventricle and into the pulmonary artery. But instead of completing the entire pulmonary circuit, the blood is shunted directly from the right ventricle into the aorta through a special fetal blood vessel called the *ductus arteriosus.*

At birth, when the baby takes its first breath, blood flow through the umbilical cord decreases and within a few minutes after birth pulsations in the cord subside. The newborn child then receives oxygen through the lungs and the vascular shunts which cause blood to bypass the lungs become nonfunctional. Soon after birth the foramen ovale closes and the ductus arteriosus degenerates.

In addition to performing exchange functions the placenta is also a source of hormones. Several of these hormones have biological effects similar to some of the pituitary hormones. For example, the placental hormone chorionic gonadotropin stimulates the ovary to secrete steroid hormones, an action similar to the pituitary gonadotropins. Placental lactogen is another hormone secreted by the placenta, the effects of which are probably to induce changes in the breasts in preparation for milk formation and also to induce changes in carbohydrate and fat metabolism. A hormone similar to pituitary thyrotropic hormone (TSH) has also been identified in placental tissue. By the sixth week of development the placenta begins to secrete steroid hormones normally produced by the ovary, estrogen and progesterone. The role of estrogen during pregnancy appears to be the alteration of the metabolic systems of the mother so that she can accommodate the demands of pregnancy. Estrogen is also probably involved in growth of the breasts and uterus during pregnancy. Progesterone is important during pregnancy for it is involved in the maintenance of a uterine lining that can allow and support implantation, and it also appears to foster the quiescence of uterine musculature during pregnancy which may help prevent uterine contractions and a possible premature labor.

CONGENITAL ABNORMALITIES

Fetal development can sometimes proceed abnormally to the degree that it results in a serious anatomical malformation of one or more of the body's organs or a biochemical disturbance that causes a metabolic deficiency. Since these abnormalities are present at birth, they are referred to as congenital abnormalities or birth defects. Estimates of the incidence of congenital abnormalities are variable, but they tend to fall within the range of between one and four percent of live births (Langman, 1969, Morison, 1970).

Congenital abnormalities can be caused by many factors. Some abnormalities are known to be associated with defects in chromosome number or structure, or the expression of particular genes on otherwise normal appearing chromosomes. Still other birth defects are caused by the harmful influence of certain environmental agents. Of the many substances a pregnant woman can take into her body or can come in contact with, such as food, additional vitamins, alcohol, drugs for medication, drugs for pleasure, cigarettes, and a variety of infectious organisms, some may be transported across the placenta and cause malformations or disease in the fetus. Environmental agents that cause birth defects are called *teratogens*. There are examples of specific birth defects—so-called phenocopies—that can be produced by either chromosomal-genetic abnormalities or teratogens.

A congenital abnormality that is associated with an abnormal number of chromosomes is *Down's syndrome* (formerly called mongolism). Down's syndrome is characterized by the presence of three members of the chromosome type numbered 21 instead of the usual two. Thus, Down's syndrome is also referred to as *trisomy 21*. Such a chromosomal aberration usually arises during the maturation of either the spermatozoon or ovum so that one of these gametes matures with an abnormal number of chromosomes (in this case two chromosome "21") which are then passed to the offspring at fertilization. The characteristic features of a person with Down's syndrome are severe mental retardation and a variety of deformities of the hands and feet. The incidence of Down's syndrome is approximately 1 in 700 births, but in children born to mothers over 45 years old, the incidence is about 1 in 50 (Morison, 1970).

An abnormal number of sex chromosomes can also produce birth defects. *Klinefelter's syndrome* is a congenital abnormality that is associated with an XXY complement of sex chromosomes, which can be produced either by the fusion of a spermatozoon with a single Y sex chromosome and an ovum with two X chromosomes or by the union of a spermatozoon with an abnormal XY pair of sex chromosomes and an ovum with a single X sex chromosome. In either case, the result is a chromosome complement consisting of 44 autosomes and an XXY set of sex chromosomes. The presence of the Y chromosome gives a person with Klinefelter's syndrome many of the characteristics of a male, but because of the additional X chromosome, normal male sexual development is deficient. The testes are small and the seminiferous tubules are undeveloped, and the person is always sterile.

Another sex chromosome abnormality is the XYY chromosome complement. The discovery of men with two Y chromosomes originally invited the hypothesis that these men would in some way be "super males" and probably overly aggressive and violent. This hypothesis was given some credence when a number of prison inmates were found to have this abnormal genetic constitution. It was later determined, however, that the proportion of men in the population at large with the XYY complement was as great as the proportion among prison inmates. It is still undetermined whether or not there is a correlation between the occurrence of the extra Y chromosome and any propensity for violent behavior.

An example of a congenital abnormality that is caused by the absence of one sex chromosome rather than one extra one is *Turner's syndrome*. People with Turner's syndrome have a sex chromosome complement consisting of a single X chromosome, a condition which is designated XO. Turner's syndrome is characterized by the absence of ovaries (and hence sterility), underdeveloped breasts, and certain skeletal deformities.

There are a number of congenital abnormalities that are genetic in origin but which are not associated with observable aberrations in chromosome number and structure. Very often these abnormalities are caused by defects in single genes, the expression of which leads to the production of abnormal proteins. This situation can result in a biochemical disturbance that is the basis of a particular disease. An example of a congenital anomaly whose basis is a defective gene is *sickle cell anemia.*

Sickle cell anemia is a disease of the blood that results from the abnormal sickling of the oxygen-carrying red blood cells. Normally red blood cells are shaped like a biconcave disc, but in persons with sickle cell anemia the shape of the red blood cell is distorted into a curved or sickle shape. One consequence of the sickling is that the red blood cells are broken down faster than normal red blood cells, which causes the anemia. In addition, the sickled cells are more rigid than normal red blood cells and tend to clog small capillaries. This prevents oxygen from reaching tissues and leads to the onset of a "crisis"—an acute episode of pain and fever. Other difficulties encountered by persons with sickle cell anemia include retarded development, jaundice, kidney disease, and an increased susceptibility to infection.

The defective gene that causes sickle cell anemia is one that codes for the chemical structure of a portion of the oxygen-carrying molecules of red blood cells, hemoglobin. Hemoglobin is made of primarily four protein subunits, two identical alpha subunits and two identical beta subunits. In sickle cell anemia, the gene that codes for the chemical structure of the beta subunits is abnormal and hence produces a pair of beta subunits that differ in chemical composition from normal beta subunits. This chemical difference causes sickle cell hemoglobin to have an abnormal three-dimensional structure which promotes the stacking of the molecules into long arrays within the red blood cells. The stacking of the hemoglobin molecules ultimately distorts the red blood cell into the sickle shape and the pathology of the disease results.

Sickle cell anemia occurs principally in black people. It is estimated that in the United States, 1 in every 500 black children is born with sickle cell anemia, and that between 25,000 and 50,000 people have the disease now. Another 2 million black people carry the gene for the disease (sickle cell trait), but rarely do they experience any symptoms of the disease. At the present time there is no cure for sickle cell anemia, and many of the people born with the disease die before they reach middle age.

In some instances it is possible to suspect that a fetus will be born with a congenital abnormality caused by a chromosomal aberration or a genetic defect. For example, older women who become pregnant stand a high risk of giving birth to children with Down's syndrome. And there are many genetic diseases—so-called inborn errors of metabolism—that can be inherited from parents who have the disease or who are free of symptoms of a particular genetic disease but who are probably carriers of the defective gene. By employing a technique called *amniocentesis* a doctor can obtain a sample of fetal cells to determine if any chromosomal abnormalities or biochemical deficiencies exist.

Amniocentesis involves withdrawing amniotic fluid from the pregnant woman sometime between the fourteenth and sixteenth weeks of pregnancy. Fetal cells present in the amniotic fluid are withdrawn along with the fluid, and these cells can be examined for trisomies or absent chromosomes, and biochemical tests can be performed to see if certain particular metabolic disorders are present. If a very serious abnormality is found, and should the parents choose to do so, a saline abortion can be performed before the twentieth week of development and the pregnancy terminated.

One of the most widely publicized teratogenic conditions is rubella infection (German measles) in the mother. Rubella is caused by a virus. Although this disease is not particularly harmful to the mother, in the early weeks of pregnancy it is known to cause serious developmental defects, mainly to the eyes, middle ear, and heart. Occasionally the infection will cause fetal death. The incidence of deformation due to maternal rubella infection is about 20 percent if the disease is contracted within the first 13 weeks of pregnancy.

An example of a chemical substance that is teratogenic is the drug, thalidomide. During the early 1960s many pregnant women in Western Europe were given the new drug thalidomide to be used as a mild sedative. Its effects upon the fetus were of course not known at that time. Eventually an increase in the number of babies born with the relatively rare congenital anomaly called *phocomelia* (a condition characterized mainly by deformities in the limbs and sometimes even total absence of limbs) was observed. An epidemiological study later showed a high correlation between the birth of a child with phocomelia and the ingestion of thalidomide by the mother during the first months of pregnancy. Thereafter, thalidomide became contraindicated for use by pregnant women.

Several chemicals in addition to thalidomide are known to be teratogenic in humans. Most of these agents inhibit the growth of cancer cells, and so it is not surprising that they are active against the dividing cells of the fetus. These compounds include aminopterin, flurouracil, and cyclophosphamide. They have been given to pregnant women usually in an attempt to induce an abortion, and when that failed, the treatment resulted in the birth of a deformed child.

Radiation is also a potent teratogen. Up to 25 percent of the children born to women who were pregnant at the time of the atomic bomb explosions over Hiroshima and Nagasaki in 1945 had congenital abnormalities.

In certain circumstances sex hormones can cause developmental defects. Administration of androgens to a pregnant woman can cause masculinization of an otherwise normal female fetus (see Chapter 2). And although a pregnant woman would rarely take androgens, there have been instances in which doctors prescribed progestational compounds to women to increase the amount of circulating progesterone in an attempt to maintain an apparently feeble pregnancy. Unfortunately these compounds were converted to androgenlike substances by the mother's normal metabolic processes and the female fetuses were masculinized. Such hormone therapy is no longer practiced.

Another teratogenic hormonal substance is stilbesterol. About twenty years ago stilbesterol was given to pregnant women in whom the normal output of estrogen during pregnancy was believed to be low. The stilbesterol, being a synthetic estrogen, was administered to bolster the low estrogen output and prevent spontaneous abortion. The children born to these mothers appeared normal at birth, but recently it became apparent that many of the daughters of these women developed a rare form of vaginal cancer. This occurrence came as a complete surprise to many medical professionals since the harmful effects of stilbesterol became evident at such a relatively late time in life. It has served to increase the caution with which doctors prescribe medication during pregnancy.

Some substances may not cause developmental abnormalities, but they may harm the fetus in other ways. For example, heroin and opium derivatives are passed by the placenta, and children born to mothers who are addicts become addicted before they are born. After birth, if they are not treated for their addiction they may experience withdrawal and may die.

A fetus can contract syphilis from its mother if she is not free of the disease after the first weeks of pregnancy. The organism that causes syphilis can get across the placenta and cause infection in the fetus before it is even born. It is estimated that 80 percent of the children born to mothers with syphilis will have the disease. Of these, more than half will die of the disease and the rest are destined to develop the symptoms of syphilis at some time in their lives (see Chapter 4). If a pregnant woman with syphilis receives proper treatment before the fourth month of pregnancy, there is a good chance that she will not pass her infection to her child.

Recent studies have demonstrated that maternal smoking during pregnancy can retard the growth of the fetus and perhaps cause premature birth (HEW Report on Smoking and Health, 1972). It is also possible that smoking mothers have more stillbirths and neonatal deaths than nonsmoking mothers.

MULTIPLE PREGNANCY

Most often human mothers are pregnant with only one fetus at a time; however, multiple pregnancies involving two, three, and as many as six fetuses do occur. The incidence of twinning in the United States is about 1 in every 100 births, whereas triplet births number 1 in 10,000. Higher-order multiple births are extremely rare. The incidence of twinning in the black population is slightly higher than in the white population, and twinning occurs least often in Asians.

Twinning results either from the fertilization of two separate ova during the same ovulatory cycle, called *dizygotic twinning,* or from a single fertilized ovum which breaks apart during the early cleavages of the zygote and subsequently develops into two nearly identical fetuses, called *monozygotic twinning.* Triplet pregnancies are rarely from a single zygote but are more often combinations of dizygotic and monozygotic twinning. Because they develop from separate ova, dizygotic twins have individual and unique genetic complements and may be of different sex. Monozygotic twins, on the other hand, are genetically identical and are always of the same sex. The frequency of births of dizygotic twins is about twice that of monozygotic twins.

Studies indicate that the incidence of dizygotic twinning is related to maternal age, the number of previous successful pregnancies, and race. Older women who have already given birth seem to be more likely to have dizygotic twins than mothers who are pregnant for the first time. And the differences in twinning frequency between the races are due to dizygotic twinning. On the other hand, the incidence of monozygotic twinning seems not to be related to any of these factors.

Conjoined, or Siamese twins, result from a single zygote in which the inner cell mass splits, but separation of the cells is incomplete and the two fetuses develop joined together. Most conjoined twins are joined back to back with part of the buttocks and sacrum in common. Other times the twins are joined at the abdomen or parts of the head. Occasionally it is possible to separate surgically the conjoined twins.

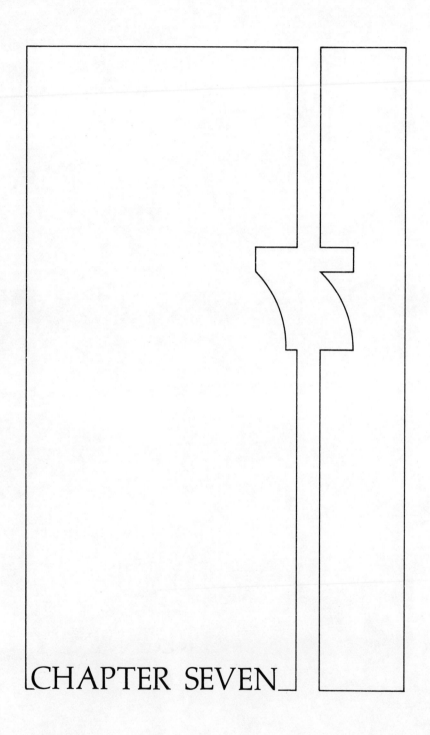

CHAPTER SEVEN

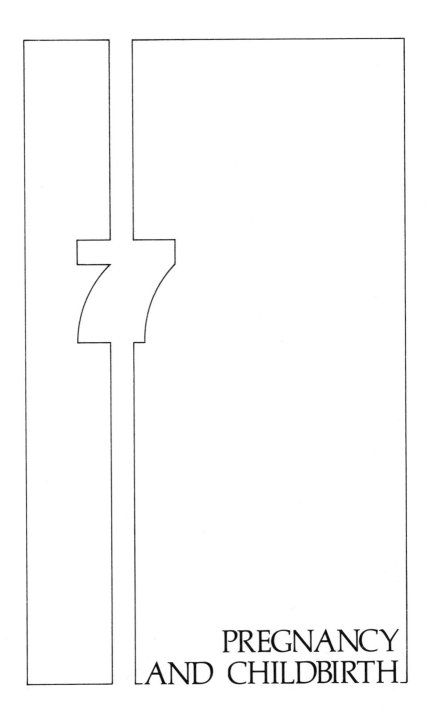

PREGNANCY
AND CHILDBIRTH

One of the characteristics of living things is that they maintain a nearly constant anatomical and physiological condition despite a continual exchange of matter and energy with their environment. Solids, liquids, and gases are taken in by an organism and utilized to provide it with both energy for metabolic and physiological activity and materials for the growth and maintenance of organic form.

When a woman is pregnant, however, a number of changes occur in her normal physiology in order to accommodate the demands of the fetus growing inside her. To comply with fetal demands for food and oxygen, the maternal cardiorespiratory system adapts to deliver these materials to the fetus. The blood plasma increases in volume to as much as 50 percent over normal levels; the heart beats 10 percent faster and with a 20 to 30 percent greater output per minute. To supply the additional oxygen needed for fetal metabolism, the mother tends to breathe more deeply and at a slightly faster rate. In conjunction with the increased intake of oxygen, there is an increase in the number of red blood cells which carry oxygen through the mother's bloodstream to the fetus developing in her uterus.

These changes in the maternal physiology are a natural consequence of being pregnant; they are the mother's way of adapting to the pregnant condition. Thus a woman with a fetus *in utero* is considered a singular physiological unit rather than two separate entities. "Pregnancy is not a process of fetal growth superimposed upon the ordinary metabolism of the mother. Fetal development is accompanied by extensive changes in maternal body composition and metabolism. . . ." (World Health Organization Committee Report, 1966). It is not necessary for a pregnant woman to alter consciously her normal daily physiological activities in order to provide for the developing fetus. In other words, she does not have to think about eating for two or breathing for two. She has the physical capacity to support the development of the fetus "naturally" through automatically controlled adjustments in her nonpregnant physiology.

One of the most striking changes to take place during pregnancy is the growth of the uterus (Figure 7–1). The nonpregnant uterus is approximately 7 cm long and weighs about 60 grams. But during pregnancy it enlarges to become approximately 30 cm long and

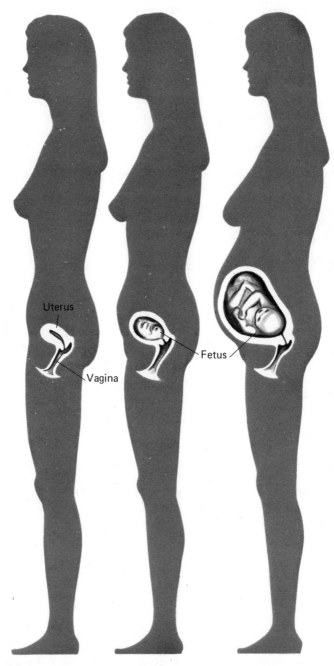

FIGURE 7-1
Growth of the uterus during pregnancy.

achieves a weight of nearly 1000 grams. Virtually all of the increase in uterine size is due to enlargement of the body of the uterus. The cervix does not grow very much during pregnancy. Uterine growth proceeds in a generally continuous fashion from the first weeks of pregnancy, but during the time when fetal growth is most pronounced, the uterus fills the entire abdominal cavity and then creates the protrusion of the abdomen that is so characteristic of pregnancy.

HORMONAL CHANGES IN PREGNANCY

Many of the changes in a woman's nonpregnant physiology to the state of pregnancy are brought about and maintained by the steroid sex hormones, estrogen and progesterone. The specific actions of these hormones during pregnancy are difficult to determine experimentally due to the complexities of the metabolic changes they control. Nevertheless, it is possible to ascribe to estrogen a dominant role in the following processes: (1) the formation of new muscle fibers in the muscular coat of the uterus to allow for expansion due to fetal growth; (2) proliferation of milk ducts in the breasts preparative to nursing the newborn; (3) increase in arterial vascularization in the uterine lining; (4) changes in a host of metabolic enzyme systems to accommodate the maternal physiology to the pregnant condition. The effects of progesterone seem to be related to the maintenance of the uterus in a condition favorable for implantation and subsequent embryonic growth. It also seems to enhance some of the effects attributed to estrogen.

During the first three months of pregnancy the corpus luteum is the main source of the steroid hormones. Near the end of that period of time the placenta gradually becomes responsible for the production of these hormones and the secretory capabilities of the corpus luteum wane. Recall that in the normal 28-day menstrual cycle the corpus luteum degenerates after a 10-day lifespan and the output of steroid hormones consequently falls off (see Chapter 5). And without the stimulatory effects of estrogen and progesterone, the uterine lining breaks up and is lost in a menstrual discharge. If this were to occur in the cycle in which fertilization took place, then the fertilized ovum and the nutritive bed in which it implanted would be shed and a successful pregnancy would have been thwarted. Thus it is imperative that the secretory lifetime of the corpus luteum be extended beyond the usual 10 days of a "corpus luteum of menstruation" to the three or so months of a "corpus luteum of pregnancy."

The change from a corpus luteum of menstruation to one of pregnancy is brought about by the placental protein hormone, chorionic gonadotropin (abbreviated HCG). HCG is produced by the trophoblast soon after the blastocyst implants in the uterus. When maternal blood vessels are tapped by the advancing trophoblast approximately 10 days after fertilization, the HCG produced by the trophoblast diffuses into the maternal blood, and when carried by the circulation to the ovaries, stimulates the corpus luteum to continue the secretion of steroid hormones beyond its normal lifetime. Thus HCG acts as a messenger from the implanted fertilized ovum to the corpus luteum notifying it that implantation has occurred and that a state of pregnancy exists. The "delivery" of this message near the end of the normal menstrual cycle is at just the proper time to prevent the degeneration of the corpus luteum and the loss of the pregnancy.

Measurements of HCG in the urine or blood of pregnant women show it to rise to very high levels during the second month of pregnancy and then drop to almost zero by the fourth month (Figure 7–2). By this time in the pregnancy, the placenta itself has grown sufficiently to be fully capable of supplying the steroid hormones necessary to maintain the pregnancy, and the stimulation of the corpus luteum by HCG to form steroid hormones falls off. Without the stimulatory effects of HCG, the corpus luteum of pregnancy degenerates, and the hormonal maintenance of the pregnancy is left solely to the placenta.

One of the consequences of the change in steroid hormone secretion during pregnancy is that normal monthly ovulations cease. At no time in the pregnancy are ova matured and ovulated. This happens because the high levels of steroid hormones in the maternal blood produced by the corpus luteum and the placenta inhibit the

149

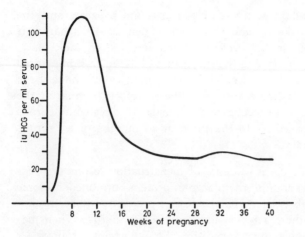

FIGURE 7-2
Serum levels of HCG during pregnancy. From F. Hytten and I. Leatch, *Physiology of Human Pregnancy*, 2nd ed. (New York: Oxford University Press, 1971). Reprinted by permission.

pituitary secretion of gonadotropic hormones, FSH and LH. Without the stimulatory action of these hormones, ovulation is not possible.

NUTRITION DURING PREGNANCY

An important aspect of successful pregnancy is the maternal diet. A mother must eat a well-balanced diet if she and her child are to be healthy. Although an increase in appetite may occur automatically as a result of the physiological adaptation to pregnancy, there is no guarantee that a mother's choice of foods will be nutritious for herself and her child. The most important dietary constituent during pregnancy is protein, for the developing fetus is continually growing by making new cells of which protein is the major solid constituent. The Food and Nutrition Board of the National Research Council recommends an increase of 10 grams daily of

TABLE 7.1
RECOMMENDED DAILY DIETARY ALLOWANCES

	Nonpregnant (18-22 yrs)	Pregnant	Lactating
Protein	55 g	65 g	75 g
Calcium	0.8 g	0.12 g	0.13 g
Phosphorus	0.8 g	0.12 g	0.13 g
Iodine	100 mg	125 μg	150 μg
Iron	18 mg	18 mg	18 mg
Magnesium	350 mg	450 mg	450 mg
Vitamin A	5000 iu	6000 iu	8000 iu
Vitamin D	400 iu	400 iu	400 iu
Vitamin E	22 iu	30 iu	30 iu
Vitamin C	55 mg	60 mg	60 mg
Folic acid	0.4 mg	0.8 mg	0.5 mg
Niacin	13 meq	15 meq	20 meq
Riboflavin	1.5 mg	1.8 mg	2.0 mg
Thiamine	1.0 mg	1.1 mg	1.5 mg
Vitamin B_6	2.0 mg	2.5 mg	2.5 mg
Vitamin B_{12}	5 μg	8 μg	6 μg
Total calories	2000	2200	3000

SOURCE   Food and Nutrition Board of National Research Council, 1962.

dietary protein during pregnancy (Table 7–1). This amounts to a total dietary intake of nearly 65 grams of protein per day during pregnancy in comparison to 55 grams a day for a nonpregnant woman. The increased amount of protein is probably most vital in the second half of pregnancy because that is the time of greatest fetal growth. Good sources of protein are meat, milk, poultry, cheese, and fish.

Many doctors suggest that a mother supplement her diet with additional vitamins and perhaps iron. The iron is deemed important because of the increased amounts of the oxygen-carrying molecule hemoglobin in both maternal and fetal bloods. There are four atoms of iron in every molecule of hemoglobin, and these are essential for the oxygen-carrying capability of that molecule.

A certain gain in weight is to be expected during pregnancy, but it is unwise to become obese. What can be expected is that by the end of pregnancy the average woman will have gained 20 to 25 pounds. Seven of these pounds are contributed by the fetus itself. The enlarged uterus accounts for an additional 2 pounds, and the amniotic fluid and placenta add 1 pound each. To sustain all of this living tissue for the duration of pregnancy, somewhere between 4 and 8 pounds of fluid are added to the maternal system, both as extra blood volume and as supplemental extracellular fluid. Some women may gain up to 4 pounds of additional body fat which can be mobilized to provide nutrient for the mother and child during brief periods of no food intake.

DIAGNOSIS OF PREGNANCY

The many changes in a woman's normal body physiology which accompany the onset of pregnancy are usually known well enough to women of reproductive age so that many women often suspect they are pregnant long before they consult a doctor for a confirmatory diagnosis. It must be pointed out, however, that most of the symptoms recognized as resulting from pregnancy may be due to other physiological conditions which do not involve the presence of a fetus growing in the uterus. Therefore all the "symptoms of pregnancy" attributed to the changes in a woman's physiology must be considered presumptive until the presence of a living fetus in the uterus is confirmed (Table 7–2).

The most commonly recognized symptom of pregnancy is a missed menstrual period. This occurs in pregnancy because implantation has taken place, and the trophoblast is producing HCG and consequently the corpus luteum does not degenerate. With the corpus luteum remaining intact and active, the levels of steroid hormones in the blood remain high so that a normal menstrual period is forestalled.

A missed menstrual period, however, can result from physiological abnormalities unrelated to pregnancy and even from psychologically upsetting experiences, such as a change in surroundings or even the fear of pregnancy itself. This is why a missed menstrual period is not an absolute confirmation of pregnancy. Some causes

TABLE 7.2
SYMPTOMS AND SIGNS OF PREGNANCY

Symptoms	Signs
Missed menstrual period	Softening of uterus (Hegar's sign)
Urinary frequency	HCG in blood or urine
Breast tenderness	Fetal heart beat
Nausea (morning sickness)	Detection of fetus—
	x-ray
	sonography

of menstrual irregularity are malfunctions in the endocrine (hormone) glands, malnutrition, starvation (including starvation diets), and a change in climate or environment. If a woman has missed an expected menstrual period, it is possible to attempt to induce menstruation by administering a sizable dose of a progestogenic compound and then withdrawing the regimen.

Other common symptoms of early pregnancy include nausea or morning sickness, frequent urination, and tenderness of the breasts. Morning sickness occurs in about half of pregnant women and can be treated with antiemetic drugs. Urinary frequency in early pregnancy is apparently caused by the increased vascularization of the uterine area, and in late pregnancy it occurs as a result of increased pressure on the bladder exerted by the expanding uterus. The breasts become tender and sometimes painful due to the proliferation of milk ducts in preparation for nursing the newborn.

An absolute diagnosis of pregnancy cannot be made by observing changes in maternal physiology alone; it demands actual evidence of a fetus present in the uterus. The most widely used diagnostic procedure for pregnancy is the analysis of a woman's urine for the placental hormone HCG. Such determinations are possible as early as the second or third week of pregnancy. A method frequently used to determine urinary HCG is the administration of the urine presumed to contain HCG to a laboratory animal. If HCG is present, the animal gives an appropriate response to the hormone. In some instances, the urine is given to rats or rabbits, in which HCG causes ovarian follicles to rupture and turn into corpora lutea. In other animal tests, a female or male frog is given the test urine; if

153

the female ovulates or the male spermiates, the presence of the hormone is confirmed.

Probably the most common technique for HCG determination, as well as the quickest, is the agglutination test based upon the immunological characteristics of the hormone. If HCG is administered into the blood of a rabbit, the rabbit's system recognizes the hormone as a foreign substance in the blood. To remove the human hormone from the blood, the rabbit produces substances which agglutinate it. The agglutinating substances are called antibodies. The basis of the agglutination test for HCG is first to obtain serum from a rabbit which contains antibodies against HCG. When this serum is combined with a sample of a woman's urine containing HCG, agglutination occurs and pregnancy is confirmed.

HCG determination is a confirmatory diagnosis of pregnancy because its presence in a woman's blood is almost invariably due to the formation of the placenta in the uterus. This means that implantation has taken place and fetal development has begun. After the fetus has developed to some degree, other confirmatory diagnoses of pregnancy are possible. An experienced person like an obstetrician can feel the enlargement and alteration of the uterus because of the growing fetus (Figure 7–3). By the fourth month of pregnancy, the fetus can often be felt moving inside the uterus.

These intrauterine fetal movements are known as "quickening," and they are familiar to most women who have experienced pregnancy. Also, during the fourth month, it is usually possible to hear the fetal heart beating. Finally, it is possible to "see" the fetus by means of ultrasound, and only in rare instances, by x-ray. The ultrasonic method is much preferred over the use of x-rays since irradiation can be harmful to the fetus.

PSYCHOLOGICAL CHANGES DURING PREGNANCY

The stringent demands made upon a pregnant woman may oftentimes change the behavioral patterns to which she and her family

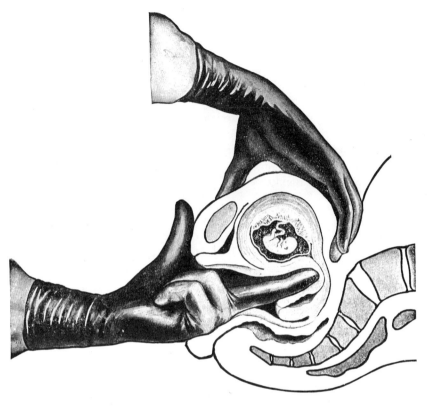

FIGURE 7-3
Hegar's sign. From J. P. Greenhill and S. Friedman, *Biological Principles and Modern Practice of Obstetrics* (Philadelphia: Saunders, 1974). Reprinted by permission.

are accustomed when she is not pregnant. A pregnant woman's emotional equilibrium may become extremely labile, with an increased sensitivity toward irritation at the slightest provocation. She may have sudden changes in mood and cry easily. The belief that all women develop some sort of "bloom of motherhood" when pregnant and are always happy is a myth; in reality, many women experience periods of unhappiness and upset during their pregnancy. This may be particularly true if the pregnancy is unwanted.

That emotional upset may occur during pregnancy must be understood by both the woman and her entire family. Indeed, many

155

doctors prefer to think in terms of "the pregnant family" instead of the individual pregnant woman, because changes in the mother's behavior will most likely affect the members of her family.

Some of the psychological difficulties experienced by some pregnant women are possibly the result of changes in the mother's physiological system. For example, the 20 or more pounds of additional weight gained while pregnant may cause considerable discomfort and make a woman edgy and prone to emotional upset. Some women are simply frustrated by their pregnancy; it may limit their movements too much, or may affect their personal appearance in ways they dislike.

It should be noted at this point that not all women have psychological difficulties when they are pregnant. Psychic changes during pregnancy are not mandatory in the way that physiological changes are. This is particularly true of women who have experienced pregnancy and childbirth previously. These women may glide through their additional pregnancies as if nothing were different. The important thing to note is that a positive attitude toward pregnancy and the desire to have the child are critical factors in making both the psychological and physiological course of pregnancy a smooth one.

Sometimes a difficult adjustment for married couples to make during a pregnancy is in the sexual relationship. Among the behavioral changes that occur in pregnancy may be the desire for sexual expression. Some women have increased sexual desires which may correspond to an increased need to be loved and cared for. On the other hand, some women may loathe the thought of sexual intercourse and abstain from sexual relations for the entire pregnancy period. Similar responses are true for husbands. Some may wish to express their joy over their wife's pregnancy by increasing sexual contact with her. Others may refrain from sexual relations for fear of hurting the fetus.

For the majority of married couples, however, it is apparent that normal frequency of intercourse is desirable during pregnancy. Long periods of sexual abstinence tend to create hardships on both husband and wife. What is not understood by many people is that sexual intercourse is not contraindicated during pregnancy unless there are signs of complications or symptoms of discomfort (Israels and Rubin, 1967). Many people are ignorant of this fact and consequently feel guilty about having sexual relations during the pregnancy period. It is probably advisable for the man to avoid putting his entire weight on the woman's abdomen during intercourse. While the woman is pregnant, the several coital positions that do not involve the man to be on top are perhaps the best to use. Very often a doctor will recommend that intercourse be curtailed in the month prior to birth and the six weeks after the baby is born. It is felt that the strong uterine contractions which accompany female orgasm might induce a premature labor, and intercourse after birth before all the vaginal tissues are healed and returned to normal may be painful and may lead to infection. Some couples find this 10-week period of abstinence centering around the birth of the child too long, in which case a doctor may deem intercourse permissible within that period so long as premature labor is not threatened and the maternal tissues are not broken (Israels and Rubin, 1967).

THE DURATION
OF PREGNANCY

The duration of the average human pregnancy is 280 days, which is 40 weeks or 10 lunar months. This is in contrast to the human gestation period—that period of intrauterine development from conception to birth—which is 266 days. This discrepancy is due to the convention among doctors and biologists to mark the beginning of pregnancy by the day of onset of menstrual flow of the ovulatory cycle during which fertilization takes place. Thus, if a woman ovulated on the fourteenth day of her menstrual cycle and if fertilization were to occur on that day, then 266 days later the baby would be born. Two hundred and eighty days is actually the average length of all pregnancies. In reality, normal, uncomplicated pregnancies can range from 260 days to 315 days. This variation is not due so much to differing gestational lengths, but is instead due to the uncertainty of the exact time of ovulation. If a woman's menstrual cycle is of an irregular length or if ovulation occurs on a day other than day 14 of the "normal" 28-day cycle, then the exact prediction of birth date is unlikely. The result is a distribution of measured pregnancy times about an average length of 40 weeks.

CHILDBIRTH

After 266 days of intrauterine life, the fetal organs which take in and transport food and oxygen—the digestive tract, the lungs, and the cardiovascular system—are fully developed and ready to assume their function independent of the mother. At this time the mature fetus is physiologically prepared to emerge from the protective environment of the uterus and face the outside world.

The termination of the intrauterine fetal-maternal relationship is referred to as childbirth, parturition, or labor. It involves the forceful expulsion from the uterus of the products of conception: the fetus, the amniotic fluid, and the placenta. The elimination of the uterine contents is brought about by strong contractions of the muscular coat of the uterus which forces the fetus and its accompanying structures through the cervix and vagina to the outside. Voluntary contractions of the abdominal muscles also help.

The entire process of labor usually takes several hours to complete, but rarely does it require more than an entire day. The time involved in labor depends, usually, upon the mother's experience with previous childbirth. If she has had children before, then her time in labor is generally less than if she is experiencing childbirth for the first time. The entire process of labor is arbitrarily divided into three stages. The first stage is the longest, lasting from eight to twelve hours in women giving birth for the first time and less time for more experienced women. During the first stage the cervix is dilated to allow for the birth of the baby. The second stage is the actual emergence of the baby and is usually of much shorter duration than the first stage. In some women, it may take only a few minutes, and for others it may require one or two hours. The third and final stage of labor is the expulsion of the placenta and fetal membranes (called the afterbirth), which usually takes only a few minutes.

The onset of labor is marked by the appearance of strong, rhythmic, and eventually frequent uterine contractions which provide the expulsive force necessary to push the baby out of the mother's body. During the last half of pregnancy, a woman may experience intermittent uterine contractions which are not associated with true labor. These are called Braxton-Hicks contractions and can be distinguished by their occurrence at irregular intervals and their rather short duration. The true contractions of labor start as roughly minute long contractions occurring at intervals of approximately 10 minutes. As labor progresses, the contractions become more intense, frequent, and of longer duration, perhaps up to 90 seconds. By the second stage of labor, the contractions occur every 1½ to 2 minutes.

The exact set of circumstances which trigger the onset of uterine contractions at the beginning of labor is still unknown. Some of the proposed theories involve changes in fetal physiology, changes in the levels of certain hormones, and stretch of the uterus and/or pressure on the cervix caused by the enlarged fetus. There is the additional possibility that a hormone secreted by the posterior pituitary gland called oxytocin is partly responsible for the onset of labor, for oxytocin can stimulate uterine contractions when administered exogenously. Whatever the cause(s), the uterine contractions of labor are completely involuntary; a woman has absolutely no control over them. They seem to occur as a result of intrinsic nervous control originating either in the muscle cells of the uterus or in the nerves of the uterine wall.

There is usually some pain associated with the uterine contractions of labor, especially in the later phases of the first stage and the beginning stages of the second. The causes of the pain are not definitely known, but they are presumably related to the stretches and strains on the uterine musculature, the cervix, and the perineum while the child is being born.

The psychological condition of the mother is vitally related to the severity of the pains associated with labor. If a woman is traumatized by the thought of an excruciatingly painful labor, then her experience may well be traumatic. Such a condition is usually the result of overstated and exaggerated stories of other women's experiences with childbirth, especially those of the mother or close relatives. On the other hand, a woman who understands and accepts the possibility that labor may be painful may actually appreciate the labor pain in her desire to participate fully in the birth of her child. There are published methods of "natural child-birth," so-called because no (or little) anesthetic or other obstetrical aid is used during labor (Lamaze, 1970; Dick-Read, 1942). These methods are based upon the mental conditioning of the expectant mother along with instruction in certain techniques of breathing and muscle relaxation which are designed to make labor proceed more easily. Occasionally hypnosis is suggested. Although not all modern obstetricians accept all the claimed advantages and proposed explanations of how natural childbirth works, many consider the idea to be quite useful. Without total dependence on anesthesia, the expectant mother will be encouraged to take a more active part in her child's birth by being conscious and in full control of her body at the time of labor.

If an anesthetic is administered in labor it will almost invariably be one that leaves the mother conscious during the course of child-birth. To remain awake is especially important during the second stage of labor when the mother must actively "bear down" and help expel the baby from her uterus. In the majority of births in this country the chosen method of pain relief in labor is the administration of a pain-relieving drug that can be taken orally or given by injection. Occasionally such drugs are given along with tranquilizers.

If pain relief is not achieved by the use of a pain-relieving drug, a doctor may decide to administer a regional anesthetic to diminish the pain associated with childbirth. These techniques involve the injection of a pain-relieving substance near the major nerves of the pelvic area. From the site of the injection the substance seeps into the nerves where it effects its anesthetic action. In one method of regional anesthesia, the anesthetic substance is injected into the lower pelvic region near the nerves which supply that region. This is referred to as "pudendal" block anesthesia, since it anesthetizes the pudendal nerve. Spinal or saddle block anesthesia is a second method of pain relief during labor. In the saddle block method the anesthetic is administered into the spinal canal where it anesthetizes the nerves of the lower spinal cord. The various methods of regional anesthesia are frequently employed because they have the advantage of leaving the mother conscious during the course of labor.

Should pain-relieving drugs or regional anesthesia provide insufficient relief from pain during labor, a mother may be brought under general anesthesia and be completely unconscious during labor. General anesthesia is applied most often in cases of difficult labor such as cesarean section, breech birth, and perhaps multiple births. Since most of the pharmacological agents which bring about complete anesthesia are freely diffusible across the placenta and therefore affect the child as well as the mother, they are used only if other methods of pain relief are ineffective.

A few weeks prior to the onset of labor, the fetus becomes positioned for its eventual birth by descending into the pelvic inlet near the cervix, a phenomenon known as "lightening." The most frequent position to be taken by the fetus is with the head nearest the cervix and the remainder of the body extended into the upper portion of the uterus. This is the cephalic or head-down presentation and occurs in 95 percent of childbirths. In the other 5 percent the fetus' intrauterine position is inverted, and the buttocks lie closest to the cervical opening or in rare instances the head-to-buttock axis of the fetus lies in a transverse plane within the uterus. In nearly all cases the legs of the fetus are folded up against the abdomen in "the fetal position."

It is fortunate that the cephalic presentation is the most common, for it allows the fetus to emerge from the uterus with less difficulty than the other less common alternatives. At the time of birth the baby's head is larger than the breech, or rump end, so the cervix must ultimately dilate to a degree compatible with the passage of the head into the vagina. Since maximal cervical dilation is needed for the head, delivery of the head first allows for the remainder of the body to follow more easily. A breech presentation would require the cervix to expand gradually as the baby emerges rather than the head-first process of expanding to a maximum at first and then gradually relaxing as the baby presents itself to the outside. It is also easier to deliver the more compact head portion with the bulky extremities coming afterward than to attempt to deliver the breech of the baby.

During the course of labor the roles of the upper and lower portions of the uterus become reversed from what they were during pregnancy. Previous to labor, the upper muscular part of the uterus expanded under the growing pressures of the enclosed fetus while the cervix was responsible for retaining the increasing weight of the fetus and placenta within the uterus. With the onset of labor these duties become reversed: the muscular upper part of the uterus contracts in order to decrease in size by expelling the fetus, and the more fibrous cervix, which was formerly rigid and strong, becomes pliable and dilated to allow for outward passage of the fetus. Before the onset of labor the cervical diameter is about 1 or 2 cm, but during labor it softens and widens to a diameter of nearly 10 cm. The dilation of the cervix is the most time-consuming aspect of labor and can sometimes last many hours.

Since the uterus, cervix, and vagina lie within the pelvic cavity, the passage of the baby out of the mother's body must be confined to the space provided by the bony pelvis. Nearly every woman is capable of delivering a normal fetus unless the architecture of her pelvis has been severely altered by injury. During a normal head-first delivery the fetus assumes a sequence of postural attitudes and positions which help it to negotiate the narrow confines of the pelvis and the curve in the birth canal.

As the fetus descends head first from the uterus under the strong rhythmic contractions of the uterine musculature, its head eventually meets resistance from the various parts of the birth canal: the cervix, the walls of the pelvis, or the pelvic floor. Having encountered this obstacle in its path, the fetal head bends forward, or flexes, so that the chin comes to lie very close to the upper chest (Figure 7–4). The importance of this flexing maneuver is that it reduces the (average) presenting diameter of the fetal head from 11.75 cm to 9.5 cm, thus making for an easier passage through the pelvic canal.

After the flexion movement the fetus undergoes a second movement referred to as an internal rotation. This movement involves a turning of the fetal head from a somewhat sideways position to one of facing front (Figure 7–5).

To this point in the delivery, the direction and movement of the fetus through the pelvic canal is downward, but since the vagina is directed toward the front of the body, the fetus must change course in the birth canal in order to be born. If this were not done, then the fetal head would continue its downward projection, and with strong enough uterine contractions, force its way out through the perineum below the vagina. Resistance to this downward movement is offered by the pelvic floor, which causes the head to move from the position of flexion to one of extension (Figure 7–6).

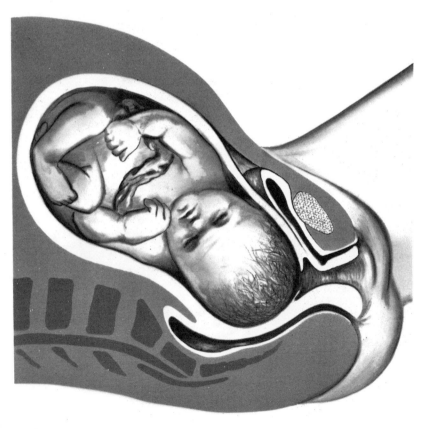

FIGURE 7-4
Flexion.

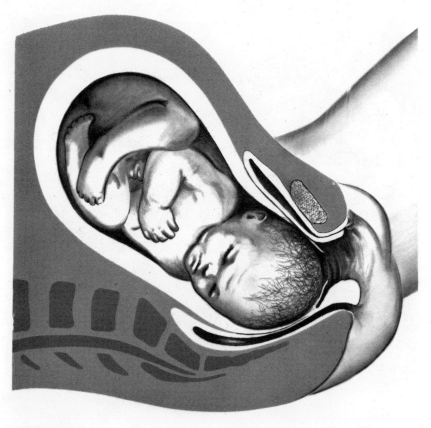

FIGURE 7-5
Internal rotation.

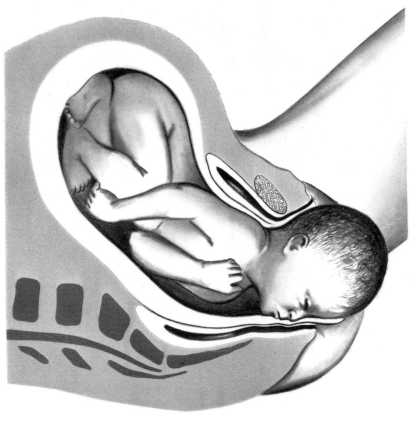

FIGURE 7-6
Extension.

The fetus negotiates the upward curve in the birth canal by the head extending in an upward direction, which aligns the direction of the movement with the vaginal outlet. With the extension of the head, the vulvar opening dilates to allow for passage of the fetal head. The head finally emerges as the top of the head, forehead, nose, mouth, and chin pass in successive order through the vaginal opening.

Immediately after its emergence, the head undergoes a second rotation which brings the rest of the body in the proper position to clear the vagina (Figure 7–7). The direction of the head rotation is sideways—back toward the side the fetal head faced before it emerged from the vagina—and it makes the delivery of the shoulders easier. The official time of birth is recorded as the instant when the entire fetal body is clear of the mother's body.

To facilitate the emergence of the baby's head at birth a doctor may make an incision in the perineum beginning at the vaginal orifice and usually extending at an angle of 45 degrees posteriorly toward the anus. This obstetric operation is called *episiotomy*. The advantage of episiotomy is that it obviates the tearing of the perineal tissues by the emerging fetus as it is forced from the vagina. A second advantage of episiotomy is that it heals much faster than perineal lacerations that might occur if no incision were made. The repair of episiotomy is usually made after the placenta is delivered from the uterus and healing requires from several days to a week or more.

Soon after the birth of the baby, the uterus begins to contract and return to its original size. The placenta, however, cannot reduce in size, so as the uterine surface to which the placenta is attached becomes smaller, the placenta becomes dissociated from the uterus. After it is dislodged, the placenta is expelled from the mother's body through the birth canal by additional uterine contractions, along with the remains of the other fetal membranes and a quantity of blood escaping from the placental site (Figure 7-8). The dislodged placenta is called the afterbirth. Delivery of the afterbirth constitutes the third and final stage of labor.

In the majority of cephalic deliveries, there is little need for obstetric assistance by a doctor or midwife, but some deliveries are especially difficult or hazardous to both mother and child, and therefore require help. Two of the commonly occurring obstetric

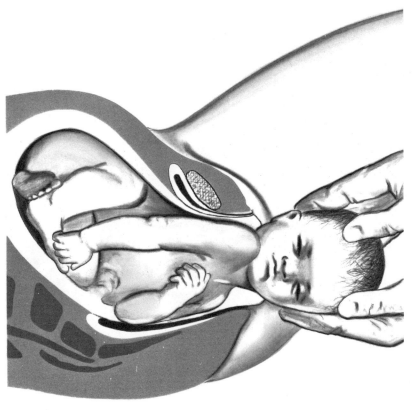

FIGURE 7-7
External rotation.

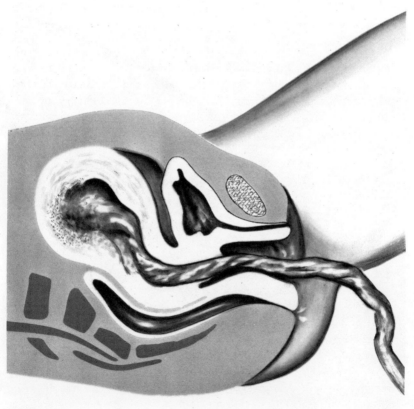

FIGURE 7-8
The afterbirth.

events which require assistance are the breech birth and the cesarean section.

In approximately 3.5 percent of childbirths the *breech*, or rump end, of the fetus is the presenting part instead of the head. The obstetric difficulties which arise from breech presentations relate to the high incidence of infant mortality caused by complications with the umbilical cord during delivery and difficulties in delivering the aftercoming head. In fact, the incidence of infant mortality in breech deliveries is many times that of cephalic births. The course of labor in breech births is dependent upon the position of the legs while the fetus is inside the uterus. A complete breech position occurs if the legs are folded up against the fetal abdomen while an incomplete breech indicates that one (single footling) or both (double footling) of the legs are extended into the birth canal. A frank breech occurs when the fetus' legs extend upward so that the feet are near the chin.

Assistance with a breech delivery is preferable after the fetus has been spontaneously delivered to the level of the umbilicus. At that point, the obstetric assistant may help with the delivery of the thorax and finally the head. The frank breech position usually acts as a better cervical wedge than the other breech presentations, but in cases where prompt delivery is necessary due to stress on the mother or child, the obstetrician may bring down both feet into the vagina and literally extract the fetus from the uterus.

Occasionally delivery through the vagina in the usual way is very difficult or even impossible, in which case the fetus can be delivered by cesarean section. *Cesarean section* is a surgical procedure in which the fetus is removed from the uterus by making an incision in the mother's abdomen and uterus. The most common reason for delivery by cesarean section is "cephalopelvic disproportion," in which the fetal head is too large in proportion to the birth canal and hence cannot pass through in the normal way. Causes of cephalopelvic disproportion are pelvic contraction and other deformities of the pelvis, or perhaps a tumor blocking the birth canal. Cesarean section may also be indicated if the uterus is dysfunctional and unable to provide contractions strong enough to expel the fetus. It is not uncommon to find cesarean section used in lieu of vaginal delivery of breech presentations in order to alleviate the possibilities of fetal death and maternal injury.

169

The cesarean section has been employed during difficult child-birth for many centuries. The origin of the name of the procedure dates from the eighth century B.C. when the emperor of Rome, Numa Pompilus, declared that such a procedure should be performed to save the life of the child if the mother were dying in labor. This law became known as "lex caesarea," caedere being the Latin verb meaning "to cut," and the operation became known as the cesarean section. There seems to be no evidence that Julius Caesar himself was delivered in this manner.

THE PUERPERIUM

After the child is born and the placenta and fetal membranes are shed, the mother enters a period of recovery called the puerperium. The puerperium normally lasts about six weeks. During the puerperium, the physiological changes brought about by pregnancy are reversed to a great degree and the mother regains her normal nonpregnant equilibrium. A fluid called lochia containing tissue debris is usually discharged from the vagina in the few days immediately after birth. The vagina and its surrounding structures undergo repair of tears, lacerations, and episiotomy if one was performed. Normal menstrual periods usually resume within six to eight weeks unless the mother is breast-feeding. The uterus returns from its 1000-gram weight at term to the nonpregnant 60-gram weight. Also during the puerperium about 4 pounds are lost in addition to the 16 or so pounds that were lost by giving up the uterine contents. This additional weight loss is due to the elimination of excess water which accrued during pregnancy as additional blood plasma and extracellular fluid. Accordingly, urine output increases during the puerperium.

An additional aspect of the puerperium is the bottle or breast-feeding of the newborn infant. The preparation of the breasts to nurse the child begins in the early weeks of pregnancy with an increased proliferation of milk ducts and the deposition of additional fat in the breast tissues. It is this growth activity which causes many women to complain of breast tenderness and even overt pain early in pregnancy. Later in pregnancy, the tenderness is likely to subside. About midway in the pregnancy the breasts begin to synthesize colostrum, a yellowish fluid which is a precursor to actual mother's milk. As the amount of colostrium increases near the end of pregnancy, it may leak spontaneously from the nipple. Due to the presence of colostrum and the concomitant build-up of breast tissue, the breasts may increase their weight by as much as 300 grams each. In addition to the growth of the breasts themselves, the nipples enlarge and often deepen in color. In blondes the nipples become a pinkish color, whereas in brunettes they become dark brown and occasionally almost black. The increased size and weight of the breasts may stretch the skin and supporting tissues of the breasts. To reduce the stretching and minimize the later sagging of the breasts after nursing is terminated, a supportive brassiere may be worn during pregnancy and the puerperium.

For the first two days after birth, colostrum is the major nutrient emitted from the breasts. Colostrum is high in protein content and is believed to give the baby some protection against diarrhea. It also contains a number of protective maternal antibodies which afford the child passive immunity against infectious diseases. As the child nurses, the colostrum is drained from the breasts and the milk ducts begin to fill with actual mother's milk.

The production of mother's milk by the breasts does not occur until after childbirth because of the peculiar hormonal regulation of the process. The synthesis of breast milk is controlled by a hormone from the pituitary gland called *prolactin*. It appears that the secretion of prolactin is inhibited by the levels of estrogen and progesterone which circulate in the blood during pregnancy. These hormones are produced by the corpus luteum and placenta for the entire pregnancy. When the placenta is expelled from the uterus in the afterbirth, these hormones all but disappear from the bloodstream and the secretion of prolactin is thereby initiated.

Breast-feeding requires the coordination of the mother and child to the degree that they become a functional unit, interdependent upon mutual contact to perform the feeding act. With the insertion of the nipple into the baby's mouth, the child instinctively begins to suck. The sucking in turn produces a nervous stimulus that terminates in the posterior pituitary gland with the release of the hormone, oxytocin. This hormone circulates through the blood to the breasts, where it effects the release of milk. This phenomenon is know as "milk letdown" (Figure 7–9).

Because the brain is central to the success of breast-feeding in both the pituitary secretion of prolactin to produce the milk and the secretion of oxytocin to effect milk letdown, it is important that nursing mothers be free from psychological adversity. Disturbances such as fear, anxiety, and pain can upset the neurological mechanisms associated with milk production and release.

A mother can nurse her child for many months. As long as the child is feeding and draining the breasts of milk, the hormonal stimulation of milk production will continue. By halting to breast-feed, the breasts automatically "dry up." If a woman wishes not to breast-feed her child, she can suppress milk production from the start by taking sex steroids which inhibit the secretion of prolactin by the pituitary.

Some women may be unable to breast-feed their children or may have to stop because of insufficient milk production or cracked nipples and instead rely on bottle feeding. Since the late nineteenth century, bottle feeding has become more and more practical due to improvements in sanitary methods and increased information about human nutrition until now approximately 80 percent of U.S. infants are not breast-fed past the age of one month (Fomon, 1967). The composition of human milk and formula-enriched cow's milk is quite similar (Table 7–3), so there is little support to the contention that breast-fed babies are nutritionally better off than formula-fed babies. To date there is no evidence to show that postnatal growth is any different for breast- or bottle-fed infants. There are certain advantages to breast-feeding which make it a desirable practice, however. Among these are the low incidence of infant diarrhea in breast-fed children and the increased immunity derived from antibodies present in the mother's milk. In addition, there is speculation from psychiatric sources that breast-feeding leads to a healthier and better adjusted later life (Applebaum, 1970).

172

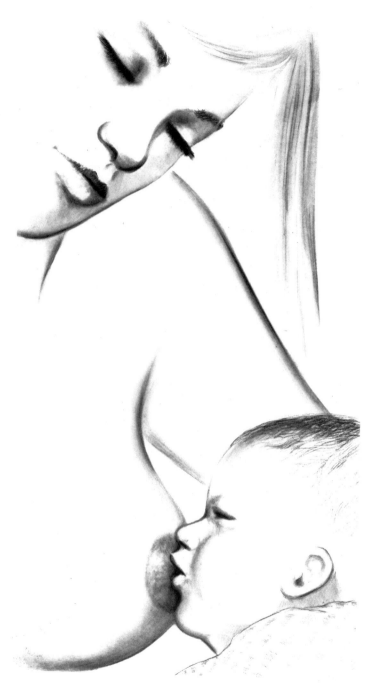

FIGURE 7-9
Milk letdown.

TABLE 7.3
COMPOSITION OF HUMAN'S MILK AND COW'S MILK

	Human	Cow
Calories (Cal/l)	747	701
Specific Gravity	1.031	1.031
pH	7.01	6.6
Minerals (g/l)		
Sodium	0.172	0.768
Potassium	0.512	1.43
Calcium	0.344	1.37
Magnesium	0.035	0.13
Phosphorus	0.141	0.91
Sulphur	0.14	0.30
Chlorine	0.375	1.08
Iron	0.50	0.45
Protein (g/l)	10.6	32.46
Carbohydrate (g/l)	71	47
Fat (g/l)	45.4	38
Vitamins		
Vitamin A (mg/l)	0.61	0.27
Thiamine (mg/l)	0.142	0.43
Riboflavin (mg/l)	0.373	1.56
Vitamin B_6 (mg/l)	0.18	0.51
Nicotinic Acid (mg/l)	1.83	0.74
Folic Acid (μg/l)	1.4	1.3

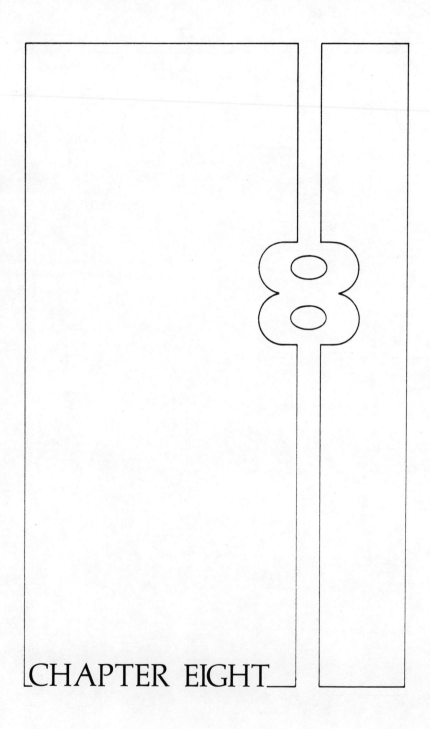

CHAPTER EIGHT

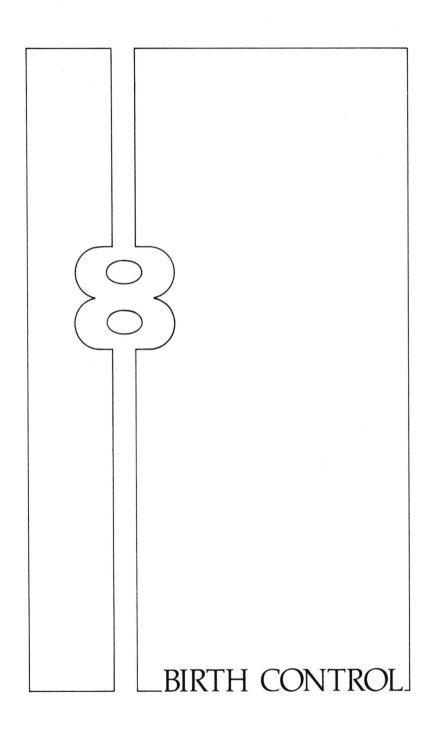

8

BIRTH CONTROL

Many people wish to exercise control over the number of children they will have and when they will be born. Some couples want to control the number and timing of the children's birth to fit their economic and psychological abilities to act as parents. They want to be sure that they are able to provide for each child's material and psychological needs without placing undue hardship on themselves or the child. Couples that are economically and psychologically capable of having many children may nevertheless choose not to produce large families or any children at all because they feel they should take some personal responsibility in limiting human population growth. Whereas at one time it might have been acceptable and even desirable to have as many as five children, many couples today feel they should limit to two the number of children they have in order to simply replace themselves rather than contribute to a net increase in the world's human population. Exercising control over pregnancy and childbirth is also desirable when they endanger a woman's life, or if there is a significant chance that the child may be born deformed.

At the present time there are a number of methods which people can use to control the occurrence of pregnancy or childbirth. Of course abstinence from sexual intercourse is one way to effect birth control. But most people are unwilling (or unable) to abstain

TABLE 8.1
THE SEQUENCE OF PHYSIOLOGICAL PROCESSES IN
HUMAN REPRODUCTION

1. Growth and maturation of ovum and sperm
2. Release of ovum—ovulation
3. Tubal transport of ovum to the site of fertilization
4. Emission of sperm from testes to penis at ejaculation
5. Transfer of sperm from male to female during sexual intercourse
6. Sperm transport in the female
7. Fertilization
8. Tubal transport of conceptus
9. Implantation
10. Fetal development
11. Birth

from participating in sexual intercourse. They prefer to experience the physical pleasure and the give-and-take of love and affection that are part of sexual contact. Rather than refraining from sexual relations, these people instead use one (or more) of the presently available methods of birth control. One group of these methods is contraceptive. They work by interrupting at some point the sequence of physiological processes and events that lead to fertilization and the implantation of the conceptus (Table 8–1). Complementing contraceptive methods of birth control are those which interrupt pregnancy after implantation has taken place but before the fetus is born. This requires the premature and artificial removal from the uterus of the developing fetus—an act known as abortion.

CONTRACEPTIVE METHODS

COITUS INTERRUPTUS

Coitus interruptus, which is sometimes referred to as the withdrawal method, is one of the simplest contraceptive practices. The procedure in coitus interruptus is simply to withdraw the penis from the vagina before the onset of ejaculation, in the belief that withdrawal before emission will prevent semen from entering the female reproductive tract where fertilization takes place. In the actual practice of coitus interruptus, the male participates in coitus for as long as he possibly can and then suddenly breaks off contact and ejaculates outside the female's body. To accomplish this feat, the male must exercise a great deal of self-control and restraint during sexual intercourse so that he can remove his penis immediately before ejaculation. Unfortunately, the control needed to practice coitus interruptus is often too demanding and the male cannot prevent himself from ejaculating inside the vagina. It is the lack of control which contributes to the fallibility of the method. Even men who can manage the ejaculatory control demanded by coitus interruptus are not entirely safe from inseminating their partner, for there is frequently a slight, unnoticed emission from the penis before actual orgasm (Masters and Johnson, 1966). Even when ejaculation does occur outside the female's body, fertilization is still possible. If semen is deposited very near the vaginal opening, it is possible that some sperm may enter the female reproductive tract. It is also possible that semen released on or near the female's abdomen or pelvic area can be inadvertently introduced into the vagina during continued sexual contact after ejaculation has occurred.

Another disadvantage of coitus interruptus is that neither partner may experience the full pleasure of sexual intercourse. When the man must concentrate on his forthcoming withdrawal, his attention is diverted from full sexual participation with his partner. This may lead to an unsatisfying sexual experience for him and also for his mate. Furthermore, many women derive great pleasure from intravaginal ejaculation; oftentimes it triggers their own orgasm. An additional psychological disadvantage of coitus interruptus that cannot be overstressed is the potential anxiety induced in both partners by the use of a contraceptive method that is risky. To await anxiously each menstrual period is certainly not the best way to carry on a sexual relationship.

THE RHYTHM
METHOD

The rhythm method of birth control is based on the fact that ovulation tends to occur near the midpoint of the menstrual cycle and that the human ovum is reproductively viable for only about two days. Hence it is reasoned that sexual intercourse will not lead to a pregnancy during times which are days distant from the most likely time of ovulation. In the regular 28-day cycle in which ovulation occurs near the fourteenth day, sexual intercourse would be regarded as safe during the days of menstruation and the few days preceding and following it, since fertilization would be most likely to occur sometime around the midcycle ovulation day.

The rhythm method is not considered to be a very reliable method of birth control. Its main drawback is that women cannot predict the exact time of ovulation during their menstrual cycle even if it is of a regular length. In a regular cycle, ovulation can occur on the day of midcycle or the day before or the day after. In cycles of irregular length, even the range of ovulatory days is difficult to predict.

For those who use the rhythm method of birth control it is often recommended that the woman keep a record of her basal body temperature in order to help determine the time of ovulation. Since there is a slight elevation in the body temperature after ovulation has taken place, a woman can keep a month-to-month record of the day of ovulation as determined by her temperature increase (Figure 8–1), and from that record attempt to predict when ovulation will occur in the next month. It should be cautioned that the recording of body temperature will only tell when ovulation *already* has occurred in a given cycle, not *when* it will occur in that cycle. Hence in any given cycle, temperature rise is most useful to determine the "safe period" for sexual relations between the time of ovulation and the onset of the next menstrual period.

Measuring the body temperature accurately requires that the woman be rested and still, preferably just after she wakes up in the morning. Too much physical activity may cause the body temperature to rise, and the results for that day be incorrect. Ultimately it is hoped that a reliable method which would allow prediction of the exact date of ovulation will be developed. Such a method would supplant the temperature method and would be a valuable addition to the rhythm method of birth control.

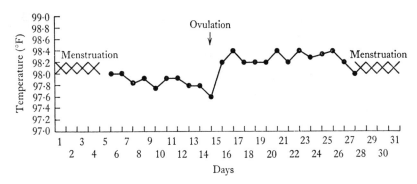

FIGURE 8-1
Graph of basal body temperature during the menstrual cycle. From J. Peel and M. Potts, *Textbook of Contraceptive Practice* (Cambridge: The University Press, 1968). Reprinted by permission.

BARRIERS TO
SPERM TRANSPORT

One of the oldest and most fundamental strategies in contraceptive practice is to place barriers between the sperm and the ovum in order to prevent their union. The barrier methods of contraception have been employed for many centuries. In an ancient Egyptian method (circa 1850 B.C.), for example, a thick paste composed of honey and crocodile dung was placed in the vagina before intercourse. A similar paste was used in India where the excrement of elephants replaced crocodile dung, apparently with equal success. In both cases, the contraceptive properties of the paste were attributable to the honey alone, which trapped the sperm before they entered the uterus. The inclusion of animal dung was to give the paste the "strength" possessed by the animal from which it came.

At the present time there are a variety of contraceptive devices in use which operate on this same strategy: they attempt to block the passage of sperm into the uterus. Some act as a physical block to sperm movement, while others are a chemical block by being lethal to sperm (spermicidal). When physical barriers and spermicides are used in tandem, they provide quite effective contraception.

A physical barrier device used by the male is the *condom,* a sheath usually made of latex rubber that covers the end of the penis and catches the ejaculate when it is released (Figure 8–2). When the condom is used properly (once only and rolled on instead of pulled on), it provides suitable contraceptive action. The use of a condom in sexual intercourse has the added advantage of providing protection against venereal disease. The failure of the condom as a contraceptive device can be attributed to the use of a punctured and therefore leaky condom, having the device slip off during sexual intercourse or after ejaculation when the penis becomes flaccid, or having the condom tear upon penetration because of insufficient vaginal lubrication. In any of these instances, sperm are likely to enter the female and the contraceptive effectiveness of the device lost.

A physical barrier device that can be used by women is the diaphragm. The diaphragm is a rubber, round, cuplike device designed to cover the cervix and block the passage of sperm into the uterus.

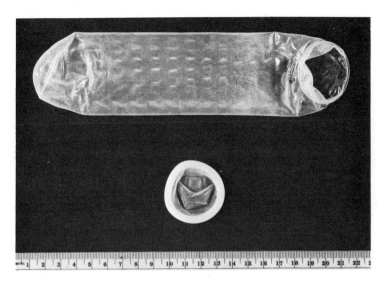

FIGURE 8-2
A condom. From H. Katchedourian and D. Lunde, *Fundamentals of Human Sexuality* (New York: Holt, Rinehart and Winston, 1973).

Before intercourse begins the woman must insert the diaphragm into the vagina. The diaphragm has a metal spring around the rim which allows the device to be folded for insertion and then return to its original shape once in place (Figure 8–3). The spring also holds the diaphragm snugly in place between the pelvic bone and the posterior wall of the vagina.

To increase the effectiveness of the diaphragm as a block to sperm movement, a spermicidal cream or jelly is placed around the rim of the diaphragm and on the side of the cup which faces the cervix. Any sperm that are not directly impeded by the physical barrier of the diaphragm will meet the chemical barrier in the form of the spermicide. When used in this manner, the diaphragm is a good contraceptive device.

It is imperative that a diaphragm fit properly. If it is too small or too large, sperm may get past the device, or it may be displaced during intercourse; therefore it is not a good idea for a woman to use a diaphragm which has not been specifically fitted for her. She should obtain her diaphragm from a doctor, who will prescribe one of proper size and also instruct in its use. In most communities, diaphragms are obtainable only from a qualified doctor.

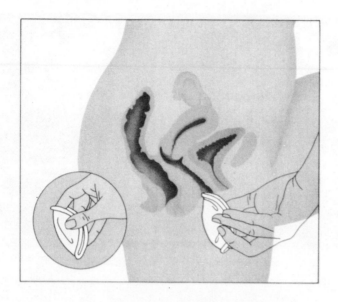

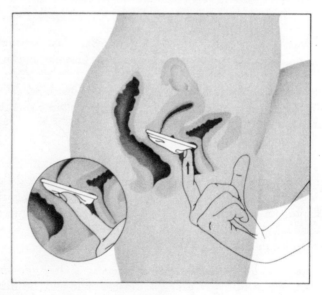

FIGURE 8-3
Insertion and positioning of the diaphragm. Courtesy of Ortho Pharmaceutical
Corporation.

A contraceptive device similar to the diaphragm in its mode of operation is the cervical cap. The cervical cap is a thimble-shaped object made of rubber, hard plastic, or metal which is inserted into the vagina to cover the cervix. To fit properly, the rim of the cap must fit snugly around the circumference of the cervix; therefore, it too must be fitted properly by a trained person.

Within recent years a number of chemical contraceptives have

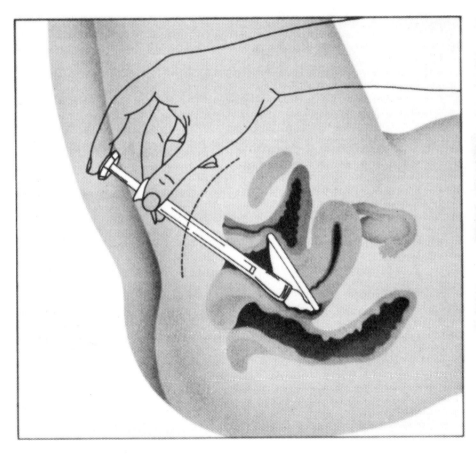

FIGURE 8-4
Application of vaginal contraceptive foam (used in conjunction with diaphragm). Courtesy of Ortho Pharmaceutical Corporation.

become available whose effectiveness is based on the ability to kill sperm. The chemical barriers come in the form of foams, gels, creams, vaginal tablets, and vaginal suppositories, all of which are applied inside the vagina near the cervix (Figure 8–4). In this position they are able to destroy on contact any sperm that are deposited in the vagina during intercourse. It should be cautioned that the contraceptive potency of the chemical contraceptives is short-lived. Although they are effective spermicides after they are placed in the vagina, their spermicidal power is diminished after a coital episode. Therefore a replacement of the original gel, cream, or foam must be made before each subsequent sexual encounter.

A contraceptive practice which has some tangential similarity with chemical modes of contraception is vaginal douching. The contraceptive power of douching is based upon the fact that douche powder and even water itself are spermicidal. This method of contraception is extremely ineffective, however, for by the time a woman can douche after intercourse, sperm are already in the uterus and on their way to the uterine tubes. It has even been suggested that the force of the water in the douche actually propels the sperm into the uterus and thereby aids fertilization.

ORAL CONTRACEPTIVE PILLS

During the 1960s there was a veritable revolution in the strategy of contraceptive practice with the advent of the anti-ovulation oral contraceptive pill, often called simply "the pill." Oral contraceptive pills were developed by Pincus and Rock in 1955, and in 1960 they were approved by the Food and Drug Administration for distribution by prescription only. Today it is estimated that nearly 8 million women in the United States use oral contraceptive pills.

The pill regimen employs two synthetic steroids which closely resemble the natural female sex steroid hormones, estrogen and progesterone (Figure 8–5). These synthetic steroids simulate the action of naturally occurring steroids which control the secretion of the pituitary hormone LH during the menstrual cycle. The eventual result of this simulation is the prevention of secretion of LH. Since LH is the hormone which induces the ovarian follicle to

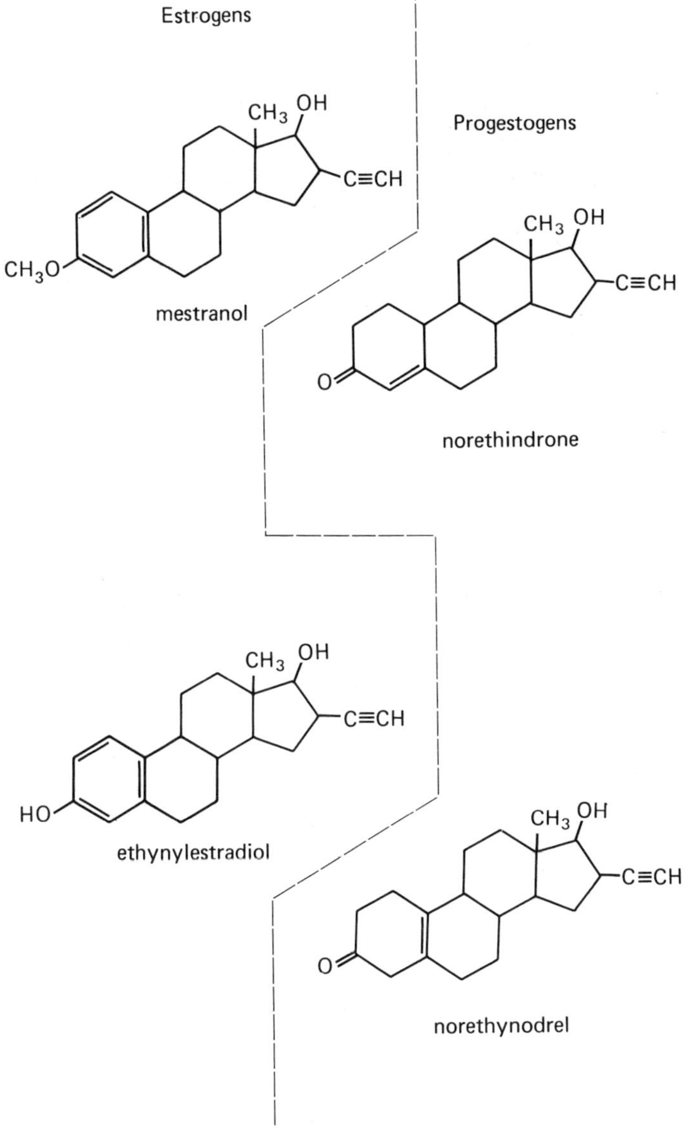

FIGURE 8-5
Chemical structures of synthetic compounds used in oral contraceptives.

rupture and release the mature ovum, inhibition of the secretion of LH means that ovulation cannot occur.

The usual regimen for oral contraception is to take one pill each day for 20 or 21 days, depending on the particular brand of pill used. Counting the first day of menstrual flow as day one, taking of the pills commences four days later on the fifth day of the cycle and continues with one pill each day for the specified time. When the pills are used up, a period of about three days elapses before menstruation begins, thus starting the next cycle. One advantage of this strict contraceptive regimen (in addition to effective birth control) is that the days of menstrual flow are exactly predictable—welcomed knowledge to women with irregular menstrual cycles.

There are presently available two classes of contraceptive pill (Table 8–2). Included in the first class are the "combination" pills. These pills have a given amount of estrogenic and progestational compound in each pill. The second class consists of the "sequential" pills. In the latter, the first 15 pills to be taken are all estrogenic with no progestogen at all, whereas the last five or six pills in the cycle are like the combination pills containing both estrogenic and progestogenic compounds. The sequential pill is designed to mimic the patterns of hormone secretion in the normal menstrual cycle, with estrogen in high amounts before midcycle and then estrogen and progesterone together in the last days of the cycle before menstruation.

Many women who take oral contraceptives experience a number of uncomfortable side effects during the first few cycles after beginning the pill. Among these are nausea, tender breasts, weight gain, and a feeling of being bloated. In most cases, these symptoms disappear after the first cycle or two, and many women are willing to put up with minor discomfort for a few weeks in exchange for the knowledge that they are free from pregnancy. Some of the other side effects of oral contraception are beneficial: they alleviate menstrual cramping in a great number of women and they afford regularity to the menstrual cycle.

Several studies have found that ingestion of oral contraceptives is related to certain serious long-term side effects (Peel and Potts, 1968). Perhaps the most publicized of these is the claim that these pills predispose a woman to the danger of fatal blood clots. These studies report that fatal embolisms, or blood clotting, occur in 1 in every 100,000 women in the population not taking oral contraceptives, while the incidence among pill takers is 3 per 100,000. What

TABLE 8.2
EXAMPLES OF ORAL CONTRACEPTIVES IN USE IN THE
UNITED STATES

Trade name	Manufacturer	Progestogen (dose)	Estrogen (dose)
Combination			
Ovulen	Searle	ethynodiol diacetate 1 mg	mestranol 0.1 mg
Demulen	Searle	ethynodiol diacetate 1 mg	mestranol 0.05 mg
Provest	Upjohn	medroxyprogesterone acetate 10 mg	ethynylestradiol 0.05 mg
Norinyl 10 mg	Syntex	norethindrone 10 mg	mestranol 0.06 mg
Norinyl 2 mg	Syntex	norethindrone 2 mg	mestranol 0.1 mg
Norinyl 1 + 80	Syntex	norethindrone 1 mg	mestranol 0.08 mg
Norinyl 1 + 50	Syntex	norethindrone 1 mg	mestranol 0.05 mg
Ortho-Novum 10 mg	Ortho	norethindrone 10 mg	mestranol 0.06 mg
Ortho-Novum 2 mg	Ortho	norethindrone 2 mg	mestranol 0.1 mg
Ortho-Novum 1 mg	Ortho	norethindrone 1 mg	mestranol 0.05 mg
Ortho-Novum 1 + 80	Ortho	norethindrone 1 mg	mestranol 0.08 mg
Norlestrin 2.5 mg	Parke-Davis	norethindrone acetate 2.5 mg	ethynylestradiol 0.05 mg
Norlestrin 1 mg	Parke-Davis	norethindrone acetate 1 mg	ethynylestradiol 0.05 mg
Norlestrin 28-1	Parke-Davis	norethindrone acetate 1 mg	ethynylestradiol 0.05 mg
Sequential Regimens			
C-Quens	Lilly	Chlormadinone acetate 2 mg	mestranol 0.08 mg
Norquen	Syntex	Norethindrone 2 mg	mestranol 0.08 mg
Oracon	Mead-Johnson	Dimethisterone 25 mg	ethynylestradiol 0.1 mg
Ortho-Novum SQ	Ortho	Norethindrone 2 mg	mestranol 0.08 mg

SOURCE   AMA Drug Evaluations, 1971.

should not be overlooked when considering these studies is the fact that fatal blood clotting occurs at the frequency of 10 per 100,000 in women who are pregnant. Thus, while oral contraceptives may be dangerous to some women, these dangers must be weighed against the dangers inherent to pregnancy. The fact that pills are available only by prescription gives doctors the opportunity to screen their patients for possible predisposition to blood clotting and thereby reduce the risk by prescribing an alternative contraceptive method more suitable to the individual for whom the pill is not ideal.

THE INTRAUTERINE CONTRACEPTIVE DEVICE

The intrauterine contraceptive device, referred to as the IUD, coil, or loop, is a device that is placed in the uterus and by virtue of this placement prevents pregnancy.

The placing of foreign objects into the uterus is an ancient contraceptive practice, known long ago to nomadic tribesmen who placed stones in the uteri of their female camels to prevent pregnancy on long treks across the desert. It was not until the twentieth century, however, that the analogous practice was applied to women in large numbers. Instead of stones, IUDs for women are made of metal, or flexible plastic, and come in a variety of shapes (Figure 8–6).

The IUD is an effective contraceptive device, but its mechanism of action is unknown. Some studies have shown that, with an IUD in place, a fertilized ovum is transported through the uterine tubes to the uterus faster than normal. This brings the fertilized ovum into the uterus before that organ is fully prepared to accept and nurture it, and hence successful implantation cannot take place. Other studies have suggested that the IUD works by creating a hostile uterine environment for the fertilized ovum. It does this by either altering the biochemical environment within the cavity of the uterus or by allowing white blood cells to accumulate on the surface of the IUD which might destroy the fertilized ovum when it arrives in the uterus.

IUDs are obtainable only from a doctor by prescription. This is to ensure proper insertion (Figure 8–7). So long as the device remains

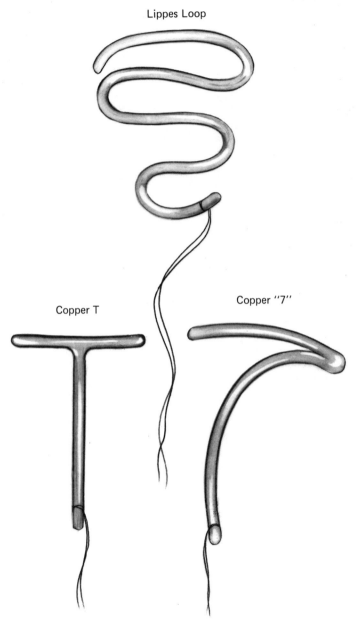

Lippes Loop

Copper T

Copper "7"

FIGURE 8-6
IUDs in use.

191

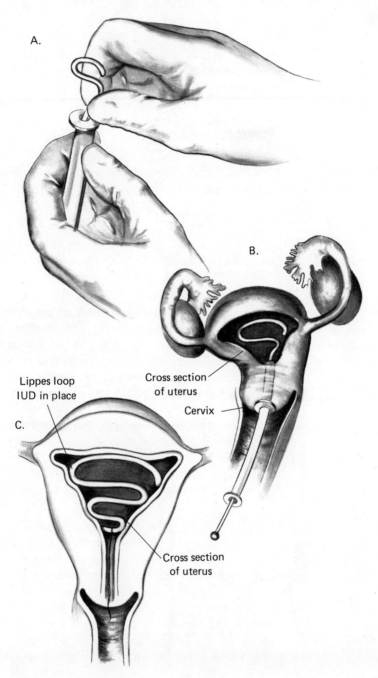

A.

B.

Cross section
of uterus

Cervix

Lippes loop
IUD in place

C.

Cross section
of uterus

FIGURE 8-7
Insertion of an IUD (Lippes Loop).

192

in place inside the uterus, its user will be free from pregnancy. There is a string attached to most IUDs which hangs down into the vagina, indicating that the device is still in place. If the IUD comes out of the uterus by mistake, which occasionally happens during menstruation for example, the woman will know it is gone and can use another form of contraception until she has her IUD replaced.

When a woman wishes to become pregnant, she need only go to her doctor and have her IUD removed.

STERILIZATION METHODS

The sterilization methods of birth control are those which attempt to terminate permanently a person's capacity for reproduction. This does not mean that a person will lose the ability to participate in sexual intercourse. Since the goal of effective contraception is to permit sexual relations without incurring a pregnancy, sterilization as a contraceptive technique must not induce the loss of copulatory functioning. The sterilization procedures currently in use include the cutting of the vas deferens in males, *vasectomy*, and the uterine tubes in females, *tubal ligation*. In certain special cases surgical removal of the uterus, *hysterectomy*, can also be performed. These operations prevent the person from contributing to a pregnancy but leave intact the person's ability to take part in sexual intercourse.

In recent years, the vasectomy has become an increasingly popular method of birth control. Fathers who decide that they want no additional children are prime candidates for vasectomy. One reason for its popularity is the relative simplicity of the operation. It can be obtained from a trained physician (usually a urologist) without hospitalization, and is performed in the doctor's office with local anesthesia in a matter of a few minutes. The operation itself consists of making an incision in the scrotal sac and then cutting the vas deferens, which is part of the sperm duct system connecting the testes with the penis. The cut ends of the duct are tied off and the incision in the scrotum repaired, completing the operation (Figure 8–8). After the operation is performed on both vasa defer-

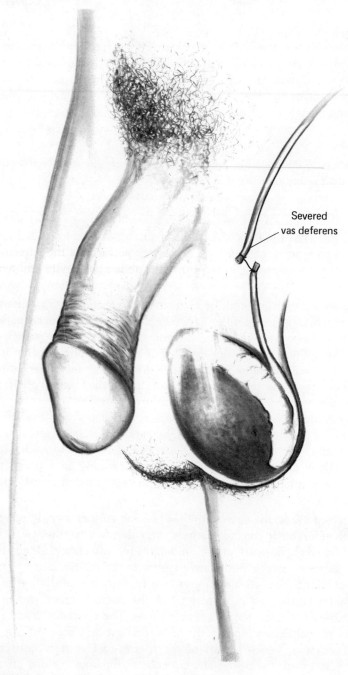

Severed
vas deferens

FIGURE 8-8
Vasectomy.

entia, sperm produced in the testes cannot pass along the sperm ducts to be emitted upon ejaculation. Their progress is halted at the tied end of the vas.

It is important to realize that vasectomy does not impair ejaculatory capacity. Since normal semen that is ejaculated is only about 1 percent sperm by volume, the other 99 percent being seminal fluid produced by the prostate gland and the seminal vesicles, the volume of fluid emitted upon ejaculation is nearly the same after the operation as it was before. The only change in the ejaculate is that after the vasectomy it does not contain sperm.

A sterilization procedure in the female which is analogous to vasectomy in the male is the cutting of the uterine tubes, called tubal ligation. This operation is not as easy to perform as the vasectomy because the uterine tubes lie within the abdominal cavity and hence are not as accessible as the vasa deferentia in the scrotum. Thus, to tie off the uterine tubes the doctor must in some way enter the abdominal region to perform the operation. This can be done by making an incision in the abdominal wall or by approaching the tubes through the vagina and uterus. Once the uterine tubes are reached they are cut and tied in a manner similar to that used in the vasectomy. And as with vasectomy, tubal ligation does not impair a woman's ability to have sexual intercourse.

CONTRACEPTIVE EFFECTIVENESS

None of the contraceptive techniques discussed thus far is ideal or perfect; all fall short of fulfilling the requirements of the hypothetical perfect contraceptive. The ideal contraceptive method should be 100 percent effective, 100 percent safe, 100 percent free of undesirable side effects, and 100 percent reversible. Furthermore, the ideal contraceptive should be easy to use and inexpensive. Some of the contraceptives presently available are theoretically 100 percent effective. Under ideal conditions or in a laboratory trial they can be found to prevent pregnancy virtually all the time. Unfortunately theoretical effectiveness is only one of the factors that contribute to the actual effectiveness of a method when it is used in the population at large. Because people do not always use their chosen method of contraception correctly, and because many of the contraceptives have inherent fallibility, the actual "in use" effectiveness of a particular method is lower than its theoretical effectiveness as determined under artificial or controlled conditions.

The use-effectiveness of a contraceptive method is usually expressed in terms of its failure rate in preventing unwanted pregnancies. The most common method of reporting failure rate is to show the number of pregnancies that would occur if the method in question were used by 100 women for a year, reported as the number of pregnancies per hundred-women-years. Using this method of measurement, the failure rates of the most commonly used contraceptive devices can be compared (Figure 8–9). The data from several studies indicate that the most effective contraceptive is the use of oral contraceptive pills, and that the IUD, condom, the diaphragm are not as effective as the pill regimen, but highly effective nevertheless. The least effective methods tend to be coitus interruptus, rhythm, and the use of foams and gels alone (Table 8–3).

The fact that the ideal contraceptive device is not yet perfected is stimulating researchers to explore alternative methods of contraception. Most of the new research is directed at exploiting pharmacological methods rather than trying to invent new physical methods. For example, there have been attempts to develop a "male pill" that would inhibit sperm production, but so far these agents have been unsuitable primarily because they also inhibit male sex hormone production, which has deleterious effects on the user's libido. Such research is continuing, however. Another direction of research involves the search for a "morning-after pill" to be taken by a woman after coitus in order to prevent any pregnancy that might have occurred. There has been some success reported with this method, using diethyl stilbesterol (DES) as the main ingredient of such a pill. Another area of investigation in the development of a better contraceptive is the attempt to exploit the immunological capabilities of women to make antibodies to sperm.

Interest in improving present birth control methods and developing newer, safer, more effective methods stems in large part from the threat of overpopulation that now hangs over the human species.

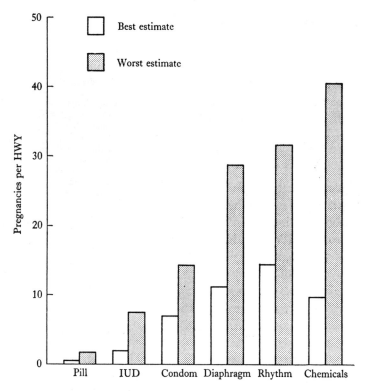

FIGURE 8-9
Comparison of effectiveness of various contraceptive methods. From J. Peel and M. Potts, *Textbook of Contraceptive Practice* (Cambridge: The University Press, 1968). Reprinted by permission.

At the present rate of growth, the earth's human population doubles approximately every 37 years. This means that by the end of this century, the more than 3 billion people that inhabit the earth today will number 6 billion. And a third of a century after that, there will be 12 billion people. It does not take a prophet to foresee that the multitude of human beings destined to inhabit the earth in the coming decades will create survival pressures on the species as a whole. There will be insatiable demands for additional food, water, space, quiet, housing, usable energy, and so forth, and governments and socio-economic systems will undoubtedly strain to keep up with these demands. Without a serious effort now to stave off increasing population pressures, the human species

TABLE 8-3
SUMMARY OF CONTRACEPTIVE METHODS

Method	User	Effec-tiveness Rating	Advantages	Disadvantages
Birth-control pills	Female	Excellent	Easy and aesthetic to use	Continual cost; side effects; requires daily attention
IUCD	Female	Excellent	Requires little attention; no expense after initial insertion	Side effects, particularly increased bleed-ing; possible expulsion
Diaphragm with cream or jelly	Female	Very good	No side effects; minor continual cost of jelly and small initial cost of diaphragm	Repeated inser-tion and removal; possible aesthetic objections
Cervical cap	Female	Very good	Can be worn 2-3 weeks without removal; no cost except for initial fitting and purchase	Does not fit all women; potential difficulties with insertion
Condom	Male	Very good	Easy to use; helps to prevent venereal disease	Continual ex-pense; interrup-tion of sexual activity and possible impair-ment of gratification
Vaginal foam	Female	Good	Easy to use; no prescription required	Continual expense
Vaginal creams, jellies, tab-lets, and suppositories	Female	Fair to good	Easy to use; no prescription required	Continual expense; unattractive or irritating for some people
Withdrawal	Male	Fair	No cost or preparation	Frustration
Rhythm	Male and female	Poor to fair	No cost; acceptable to Roman Catholic Church	Requires signifi-cant motivation, cooperation, and intelligence; useless with irre-gular cycles and during postpartum period
Douche	Female	Poor	Inexpensive	Inconvenient; possibly irritating

SOURCE H. Katchedourian and D. Lunde, *Fundamentals of Human Sexuality* (New York: Holt, Rinehart and Winston, 1973), p. 145.

courts disaster. For this reason there is a growing interest among medical researchers to produce improved birth control methods.

ABORTION

The artificial and premature termination of pregnancy is called abortion. In contrast to contraception, which aims to prevent fertilization and implantation, abortion is a method of birth control that prevents the birth of a child after the fertilized ovum has implanted in the uterus.

The removal of the fetus before birth to prevent the birth of an unwanted child is the oldest and most common method of birth control. Abortion-inducing techniques have been found recorded in ancient Chinese medical writing believed to be over 4000 years old. Hippocrates, Aristotle, and Plato all recommended abortion as a way to limit family size. A cross-cultural study found that all but one of the 300 societies surveyed used abortion as a means of birth control (Devereaux, 1955).

METHODS OF
ABORTION

There are several nonmedical methods that are used to induce an abortion. Many of them require that the pregnant woman experience some violent physical strain in an attempt to bring on premature labor and expel the fetus from the uterus. Such efforts might be lifting a heavy load, climbing trees, jumping from high places, or pressing on the abdomen. Other means to induce premature labor include stuffing foreign objects into the uterus. In nonindustrial societies, such objects are sticks, rocks, and leaves while in more industrialized societies women make use of spoons, bottles, knitting needles, and coathangers. Another technique for inducing an abortion is to place an abortifacient liquid in the uterus. Such a liquid may be made from certain herbs or the secretions of insects and other animals according to ancient prescription, or it may come directly from a bottle of industrial chemical or household disinfectant. While it is true that these vigorous methods occasionally succeed in terminating the pregnancy, they oftentimes take their toll on the mother by causing hemorrhage, shock, infection, permanent impairment of reproductive capacity, and sometimes death.

Modern medical science has evolved safe and reliable surgical abortion techniques. The most common method of surgical abortion is the *dilatation and curettage*, or "D and C" for short. This is a standard gynecological operation which is relatively simple and safe when performed by a trained person. The D and C is a two-part operation, consisting first of the dilatation of the cervix with a graduated series of dilators, each one larger than the last. The dilators are placed into the narrow cervix to wedge it open so the contents of the uterus can be removed easily. The insertion of the next largest dilator forces the cervical opening to enlarge that much more until it is large enough for the completion of the operation. Once the cervix is dilated, a curette, which is a scraping instrument with a sharp edge, is inserted into the uterus and the contents are scraped away.

In recent years a variation of the D and C has been introduced which makes use of a suction device in place of the surgical curette. Dilatation of the cervix is still a necessary aspect of the operation, but instead of scraping the uterus clean of the products of conception, they are drawn out by means of a suction aspirator. The use of suction curettage is rapidly replacing surgical curettage as the preferred abortion technique, because it is faster and presents fewer postoperative complications.

As in any surgical procedure, abortion carries some risk to the patient. One possible complication is perforation of the uterus, but this event is rare, particularly when vacuum curettage is used. Some of the postoperative complications include infection and hemorrhage, but the risk of these complications is reduced considerably when the operation is performed before the twelfth week of pregnancy.

There has been a great deal of consideration given to the psychological effects resulting from abortion. The consideration seems to center around the occurrence of postabortal guilt, depression, loss of "feminine identity," and general emotional upheaval. For many years it was tacitly assumed that having an abortion produced undesirable and occasionally severe psychological aftereffects. And whereas this view is still held by many medical and nonmedical people alike, actual studies of the psychological effects of abortion show this opinion to be unfounded. When carefully controlled psychological evaluation of women who obtained abortions is made, the finding in most cases is that there may be some guilt afterward, almost always relief, and no long-lasting psychological damage (Peel and Potts, 1968). Confirmation of the finding that abortion is rarely psychologically harmful to normal women comes from opinions of clinical psychologists and psychiatrists themselves. In a poll of mental health professionals, nearly all the respondents indicated that they rarely encountered serious psychiatric illness in their patients following abortion. Those who had encountered postabortal psychological problems often felt that the illness would have occurred even if the abortion had not taken place (Kummer, 1970).

THE MORALITY
AND LEGALITY
OF ABORTION

The propriety of abortion as a socially sanctioned method of birth control is presently under debate in the United States, although it is acceptable in other countries such as Japan, Sweden, and Hungary. Abortion in the United States first became illegal in the 1830s; then it was permitted only to save the life of the mother. Within the recent past, the abortion laws of some states had been revised to allow the termination of pregnancy if the mother's health were jeopardized (including her mental health) or if there were a significant probability that the child would be born deformed, such as the case of the mother contracting German measles during pregnancy. Some states even revised their abortion laws to allow abortion to be performed in all cases so long as the pregnancy had not passed the twentieth week and if the operation were conducted by a licensed physician. But, in January of 1973 the United States

Supreme Court ruled that no state can restrict the right of a woman to obtain an abortion within the first 12 weeks of pregnancy. Thus, at the present time the decision to have an abortion during the first trimester of pregnancy lies solely with the woman and her doctor.

Since the question of whether abortion constitutes murder is a central issue in debates over abortion legislation, many people feel that what is required is an acceptable definition of when the fetus becomes a human being endowed with protection under the law. Modern man is not the first to ponder this dilemma. Aristotle argued that the fetus possessed a soul 40 days after conception; Plato felt that a human life did not begin until birth. Many have taken the time of the fetus' first movements inside the uterus—the so-called quickening—as the time when the unborn child is a human person. Currently many people consider a person's life to begin at the moment of conception when the new individual's unique genetic composition becomes fixed.

It is important to realize, however, that all attempts to set a particular time as the beginning of a human life are completely arbitrary. From the time of the differentiation of the sperm and ovum that fuse at fertilization to the time of that child's growth to adulthood, the individual is in a constant state of change, perhaps best described as a state of becoming. To label a specific moment along this development continuum as the beginning of the human life is completely a matter of personal choice. To rationalize an abortion decision by defining some arbitrary time before which the fetus is not human only leads to further disagreement and debate.

Far more realistic in making an abortion decision are considerations about the quality of life of the unborn child and its parents. The threat of overpopulation lends striking support to women who choose not to carry their pregnancy to term. It hardly makes sense to legislate more people into a world that cannot support them. A second factor in an abortion decision is the desire to bring a child into a family that is economically and psychologically ready to receive it. The stresses of material want have an obvious deleterious effect on any child. Recent studies conducted in Sweden on children born into families that did not want them (those in which requests for abortion were denied) showed the unwanted children to have significantly more emotional problems than children born into expectant families (Table 8–4).

TABLE 8.4

FOLLOW-UP OF CHILDREN BORN TO WOMEN REFUSED LEGAL TERMINATION OF PREGNANCY

	Children born to women refused legal abortions (120)	Control Group (120)	Statistical probability
Attended psychiatric clinic	34	18	0.01
Delinquency	22	10	0.05
Drunken misconduct	19	13	0.5
Public assistance	17	3	0.001
Educationally subnormal, attended special schools, etc.	13	6	0.01
Proceeded to higher education	17	40	0.001
University	5	11	(not sig.)
Unfit for military service	60	4	0.1
Married before 21	20	14	(not sig.)
Divorced	2	0	
Girls having children before age 21	14	7	

SOURCE   H. Forssman and I. Thuwe, "One hundred and twenty children born after application for therapeutic abortion refused," *Acta Psychiatric Scandinavia*, 42: 71 (1966).

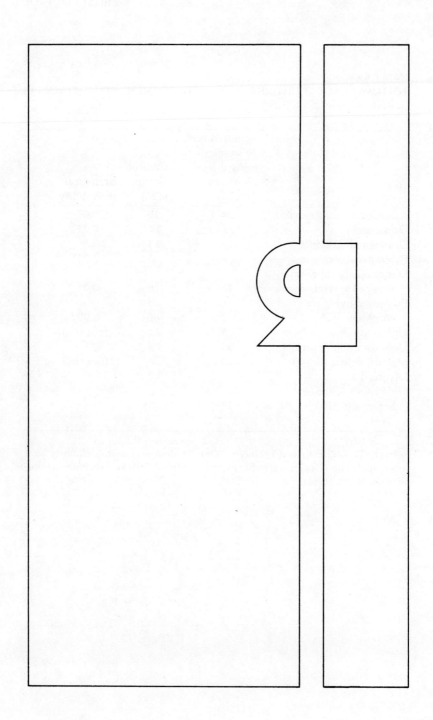

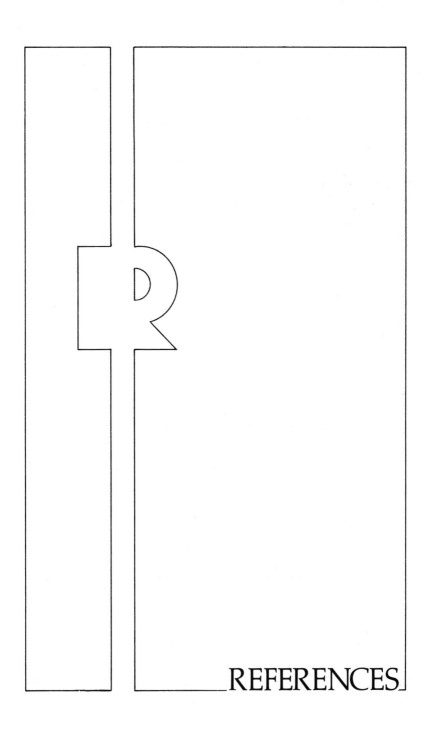

REFERENCES

Applebaum, R. 1970.
"Modern Management of Successful Breast Feeding." *Pediatric Clinics of North America*, 17:203.

Arey, L. 1965.
Developmental Anatomy, 7th ed. Philadelphia: Saunders.

Assali, N. (Ed.). 1969.
Biology of Gestation, Vols. I & II. New York: Academic.

Barnes, A. 1968.
Intrauterine Development. Philadelphia: Lea & Febiger.

Beck, M., and C. Reiterman (Eds.). 1971.
"The Destiny of the Unwanted Child." *Abortion and the Unwanted Child*. New York: Springer-Verlag.

Behrman, S., and R. Kistner. 1968.
Progress in Infertility. Boston: Little, Brown.

Bernard, J. 1970.
"Infidelity: Some Moral and Social Issues." *Science and Psychoanalysis*, 16:99.

Berne, E. 1970.
Sex in Human Loving. New York: Simon and Schuster.

Bloom, W., and D. Fawcett. 1968.
A Textbook of Histology. Philadelphia: Saunders.

Bonime, W. 1969.
"Masturbatory Fantasies & Personality Functioning." *Science and Psychoanalysis*, 15:32.

Caplan, G. 1963.
"Psychological Aspects of Pregnancy." In *The Psychological Basis of Medical Practice*, H. Lief (Ed.). New York: Hoeber Medical Division, Harper & Row.

Charney, C., R. Suarez, and N. Sadoughi. 1970.
"Castration in the Male." *Medical Aspects of Human Sexuality*, 4:80.

Churchill, W. 1967.
Homosexual Behavior Among Males. New York: Hawthorn Books.

Cleary, R., and R. Dajani. 1970.
"Current Status of Oral Contraceptives." *Medical Clinics of North America*, 54:163.

Dalton, K. 1964.
The Premenstrual Syndrome. Springfield, Ill.: Thomas.

Dalton, K. 1971. "Prospective Study into Puerperial Depression."
British Journal of Psychiatry, 118:689.

Danforth, D. (Ed.). 1965.
Textbook of Obstetrics and Gynecology. New York: Hoeber Medical Division, Harper & Row.

Demarest, R., and J. Sciarra. 1969.
Conception, Birth and Contraception. New York: McGraw-Hill.

Devereaux, G. 1955.
A Study of Abortion in Primitive Societies. New York: Julian Press.

Dick-Read, G. 1942.
Childbirth Without Fear. New York: Harper.

Drellich, M., and S. Waxenberg. 1966.
"Erotic and Affectional Components of Female Sexuality." *Science and Psychoanalysis,* 10:45.

Eastman, N., and L. Hellman. 1966.
William's Obstetrics, 13th ed. New York: Appleton-Century-Crofts.

Finch, B., and H. Green. 1963.
Contraception Through the Ages. Springfield, Ill.: Thomas.

Firth, R. 1970.
"The Social Images of Man and Woman." *J. Biosocial Science Supplement,* 2:1.

Fomon, S. 1967.
Infant Nutrition. Philadelphia: Saunders.

Food and Nutrition Board. 1968.
"Recommended Dietary Allowances," 7th ed. Washington, D.C.: National Academy of Sciences and National Research Council Publication Number 1694.

Ford, C. S., and F. A. Beach. 1951.
Patterns of Sexual Behavior. New York: Harper & Row.

Forssman, H., and I. Thuwe. 1966.
"One Hundred and Twenty Children Born After Application for Therapeutic Abortion Refused." *Acta Psychiatric Scandinavia,* 42:71.

Gorbman, A., and H. Bern. 1962.
Comparative Endocrinology. New York: Wiley.

Greenhill, J., and S. Friedman. 1974.
Biological Principles and Modern Practice of Obstetrics. Philadelphia: Saunders.

Grobstein, C. 1959.
"Differentiation of Vertebrate Cells." In *The Cell*, Vol. I, J. Brachet and A. Mirsky (Eds.). New York: Academic.

Group for Advancement of Psychiatry (G.A.P.). 1970.
The Right to Abortion. New York: Scribner.

Hafez, E. 1973.
"Transport of Spermatozoa in the Female Reproductive Tract." *American Journal of Obstetrics and Gynecology*, 115:703.

Hamilton, W., and N. Mossman. 1972.
Human Embryology, 4th ed. Baltimore: Williams & Wilkins.

Hampson, J. L., and J. G. Hampson. 1961.
"The Ontogenesis of Sexual Behavior in Men." In *Sex and Internal Secretions*, W. Young (Ed.). Baltimore: Williams & Wilkins.

Hardin, G. 1971.
"We Need Abortion for the Children's Sake." In *Abortion and the Unwanted Child*, C. Reiterman (Ed.). New York: Springer-Verlag.

Hellman, L., and I. Pritchard. 1971.
William's Obstetrics, 14th ed. New York: Appleton-Century-Crofts.

Hollinshead, W. 1967.
Textbook of Anatomy, 2nd ed. New York: Harper & Row.

Hsu, T., and K. Benirschke. 1967.
An Atlas of Mammalian Chromosomes. New York: Springer-Verlag.

Hytten, F., and I. Leitch. 1964.
Physiology of Human Pregnancy. Oxford: Blackwell.

Israels, S., and I. Rubin. 1967.
"Sexual Relations During Pregnancy and the Post-Delivery Period." *Siecus Study Guide 6*. New York: Sex Information & Education Council of U.S.

Jost, A. 1972.
"A New Look at the Mechanisms Controlling Sex Differentiation in Mammals." *Johns Hopkins Medical Journal*, 130:38.

Katchadourian, H., and D. Lunde. 1973.
Fundamentals of Human Sexuality. New York: Holt, Rinehart and Winston.

Kinch, R. 1967.
"Painful Coitus." *Medical Aspects of Human Sexuality,* 1:6.

Kinsey, A., W. Pomeroy, and C. Martin. 1948.
Sexual Behavior in the Human Male. Philadelphia: Saunders.

Kinsey, A., W. Pomeroy, C. Martin, and P. Gebhard. 1953.
Sexual Behavior in the Human Female. Philadelphia: Saunders.

Kirkendall, L., and I. Rubin. 1969.
"Sexuality & The Life Cycle." *Siecus Study Guide 8.* New York: Sex Information and Education Council of U.S.

Kummer, J. 1970.
"A Psychiatrist's View." In *Abortion in a Changing World,* R. Hall (Ed.). New York: Columbia University Press.

Lamaze, F. 1970.
Painless Childbirth. Chicago: Regnery.

Langman, J. 1969.
Medical Embryology. Baltimore: Williams & Wilkins.

Lehrman, R. 1967.
The Reproduction of Life. New York: Bantam Books.

Lewis, J. 1969.
"Impotence as a Reflection of Marital Conflict." *Medical Aspects of Human Sexuality,* 3:73.

Marmor, J. (Ed.). 1965.
Sexual Inversion. New York: Basic Books.

Marmor, J. 1969.
"Sex for Non-Sexual Reasons." *Medical Aspects of Human Sexuality,* 3:8.

Marmor, J. 1969.
Discussion of "Masturbatory Fantasies & Personality Functioning," W. Bonime (Ed.). *Science & Psychoanalysis,* 15:32.

Masters, W., and V. Johnson. 1966.
Human Sexual Response. Boston: Little, Brown.

Masters, W., and V. Johnson. 1970.
Human Sexual Inadequacy. Boston: Little, Brown.

Money, J. 1961.
"Sex Hormones & Other Variables in Human Eroticism." In *Sex and Internal Secretions*, W. Young (Ed.). Baltimore: Williams & Wilkins.

Money, J. 1965.
"Hormones in Sexual Behavior." *Annual Review of Medicine*, 16:67.

Money, J. 1965.
"Sex Errors of the Body." In *Individual, Sex & Society*. C. Broderick (Ed.). Baltimore: Johns Hopkins Press.

Money, J. 1970.
"Sexual Dimorphism and Homosexual Gender Identity." *Psychological Bulletin*, 74:425.

Money, J., and A. Ehrhardt. 1972.
Man and Woman, Boy and Girl. Baltimore: Johns Hopkins Press.

Moos, R. 1968.
"Development of a Menstrual Distress Questionnaire." *Psychosomatic Medicine*, 30:853.

Morris, D. 1969.
The Naked Ape. New York: McGraw-Hill.

Morison, J. 1970.
Foetal and Neonatal Pathology. New York: Appleton-Century-Crofts.

Pasnau, R. 1969.
"Psychosomatic Aspects of Menstrual Disorders." *Clinical Obstetrics and Gynecology*, 12:724.

Patten, B. 1964.
Foundations of Embryology. New York: McGraw-Hill.

Patten, B. 1968.
Human Embryology. New York: McGraw-Hill.

Peel, J., and M. Potts. 1969.
Textbook of Contraceptive Practice. Cambridge: Cambridge University Press.

Pomeroy, W. 1968.
"Homosexuality, Transvestism & Transsexualism." In *Human Sexuality in Medical Education and Practice*, C. Vincent (Ed.). Springfield, Ill.: Thomas.

Reid, D., K. Ryan, and K. Benirschke. 1972.
Principles & Management of Human Reproduction. Philadelphia: Saunders.

Reiss, I. 1969.
"Premarital Sexual Standards." In *Individual, Sex, & Society,* C. Broderick (Ed.). Baltimore: Johns Hopkins Press.

Rubin, I. 1965.
"Homosexuality." *Siecus Study Guide 2.* New York: Sex Information & Education Council of U.S.

Ryan, K. 1972.
"The Endocrine and Neuroendocrine Control of Reproduction." In *Principles and Management of Human Reproduction,* D. Reid, K. Ryan, and K. Benirschke (Eds.). Philadelphia: Saunders.

Saghir, M., E. Rubins, and B. Walbran. 1969.
"Homosexuality." *Archives of General Psychiatry,* 21:219.

Santamaria, B. 1969.
"Dysmenorrhea." *Clinical Obstetrics and Gynecology,* 12:708.

Sawin, C. 1969.
The Hormones. Boston: Little, Brown.

Sheinfeld, A. 1965.
Your Heredity & Environment. Philadelphia: J. B. Lippincott.

Sherfey, M. J. 1966.
"The Evolution & Nature of Female Sexuality in Relation to Psychoanalytic Theory." *Journal of American Psychoanalytic Association,* 14:28.

Shuttleworth, F. 1959.
"A Biosocial & Developmental Theory of Male & Female Sexuality." *Marriage & Family Living.* 22, 163 (1959).

Simpson, G., and W. Beck. 1965.
Life, 2nd ed. New York: Harcourt, Brace & World.

Stern, C. 1960.
Principles of Human Genetics, 2nd ed. San Francisco: Freeman.

Stoller, R. 1968.
Sex and Gender. New York: Science House.

Tanner, J. 1968.
"Earlier Maturation in Man." *Scientific American,* 218:21.

Taymor, M. 1969.
The Management of Infertility, Springfield, Ill.: Thomas.

Tietze, C., and S. Lewit. 1969.
"Abortion." *Scientific American*, 220:21.

Tietze, C. 1970.
"Relative Effectiveness of Contraceptive Methods." In *Manual of Family Planning & Contraceptive Practice*, M. Calderone (Ed.). Baltimore: Williams & Wilkins.

"Today's V.D. Control Problem." 1973.
American Social Health Association.

Turner, C., and J. Bagnara. 1971.
General Endocrinology, 5th ed. Philadelphia: Saunders.

U.S. Public Health Service Report of the Surgeon General. 1972.
"The Health Consequences of Smoking." Washington, D.C.: U.S. Department of Health, Education, and Welfare.

Vincent, C. 1968.
Human Sexuality in Medical Education and Practice. Springfield, Ill.: Thomas.

Walter, G. 1970.
"Psychologic and Emotional Consequences of Elective Abortion." *Obstetrics & Gynecology*, 36:482.

Westoff, L., and C. Westoff. 1971.
From Now to Zero. Boston: Little, Brown.

Weisz, P. 1967. *The Science of Biology*, 3rd ed. New York: McGraw-Hill.

Yalom, I., D. Lunde, R. Moos, and D. Hamburg. 1968.
"Postpartum Blues Syndrome." *Archives of General Psychiatry*, 18:16.

Young, W. 1961.
Sex and Internal Secretions. Baltimore: Williams & Wilkins.

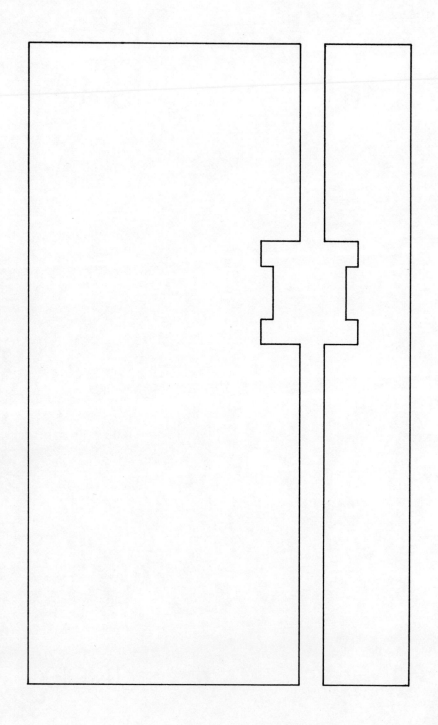

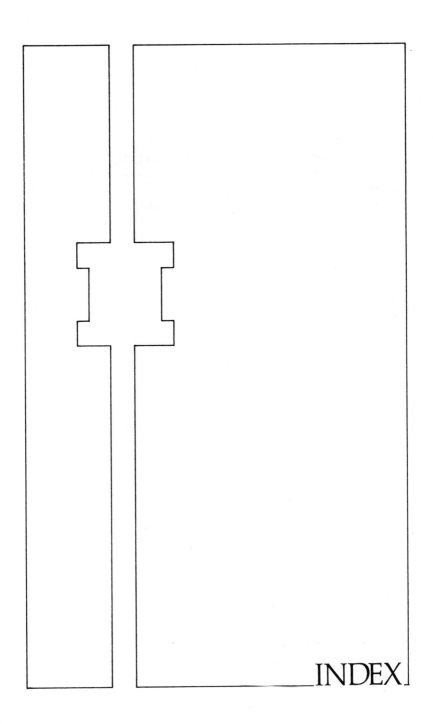

INDEX